Medicine in Virgini∶

Thomas Proctor Hughes

Alpha Editions

This edition published in 2022

ISBN : 9789356895140

Design and Setting By
Alpha Editions
www.alphaedis.com
Email - info@alphaedis.com

Contents

CHAPTER ONE

European Background and Indian Counterpart to Virginia Medicine

EUROPEAN BACKGROUND

The origins of medical theory and practice in this nation extend further than the settlement at Jamestown in 1607. Jamestown was a seed carried from the Old World and planted in the New; medicine was one of the European characteristics transmitted with the seed across the Atlantic. In the process of transmission changes took place, and in the New World medicine adapted itself to some circumstances unknown to Europe; but the contact with European developments in theory and practice was never—and is not—broken.

Because of this relationship between European and American medicine, an acquaintance with seventeenth-century European medicine makes it possible to give additional support to some of the information in the early sources about medicine in colonial Virginia. In addition, knowledge of the European background allows reasonable speculation as to what happened in Virginia when the early sources are silent.

In discussing the background for American medicine it is not necessary to make a firm distinction between England and the rest of Europe. As today, science—in this case, medical science—frequently ignored national boundaries. The same theories relative to the structure of the body (anatomy), to the functions of the organs and parts of the body (physiology), and to other branches of medical science were common to England and Europe. Medical practice, like theory, varied but in detail from nation to nation in Western Europe.

Seventeenth-century Europe relied heavily upon ancient authority in the realm of medical theory. The European and colonial Virginia physician, surgeon, and even barber (when functioning as a medical man) consciously or unconsciously drew upon, or practiced according to, theories originated or developed by Hippocrates (460-377 B.C.) and Galen (131-201 A.D.). Hippocrates is remembered not only for his emphasis upon ethical practices but also for his inquiring and scientific spirit, and Galen as the founder of experimental physiology and as the formulator of ingenious medical theories. Most often Hippocrates was studied in Galen's commentaries.

No longer do scholars or physicians scoff at the ancient authorities who dominated medical thinking for so many centuries. The seventeenth-century physician striving to reduce the frightful inroads that disease made into the colony at Jamestown may have been handicapped by the erroneous doctrines of the gossamer-fine *a priori* speculation of Galen, but the physicians to a large extent practiced according to a science rather than to superstition and magic—because the voluminous writings of Galen survived the centuries. Nor would the European physician, or his Virginia counterpart, have demonstrated the same appreciation for close observation if Hippocrates had not still been an influence.

In the realm of pathology (the nature, causes, and manifestations of disease) the humoral theory, with its many variations, was extremely popular. The humoral doctrines stemming largely from Hippocrates were made elaborate by Galen but were founded upon ideas even more ancient than either thinker and practitioner. As understood by the seventeenth-century man of medicine, the basic ideas of the humoral theory were the four elements, the four qualities, and the four humors. The elements were fire, air, earth, and water; the four qualities were hot, cold, moist, and dry; and the four humors were phlegm, black bile, yellow bile, and blood. From these ideological building stones a highly complex system of pathology developed; from it an involved system of treatment originated. In essence the practitioner of the humoral school attempted to restore the naturally harmonious balance of elements, qualities, and humors that had broken down and caused disease or pain.

The seventeenth-century, however, witnessed in medicine the trend, manifest then in so many fields of thought, away from an uncritical acceptance of the authority of the past. It also saw a defiant denial of ancient authority among those more radically inclined, such as the disciples of the sixteenth-century alchemist and physician, Paracelsus. Although some of his practices and teachings were based on the supernatural, Paracelsus stressed observation and the avoidance of a mere system of book-learning.

Practice lagged behind new scientific theory in medicine but Virginia must have felt at least the reverberations caused by the clash of the ancient and the new.

An important new school of medical theory was the iatrophysical or iatromathematical (*iatros* from the Greek—physician). This medical theory—as is the case with many scientific theories-was borrowed from another branch of science. The seventeenth century, the age of Isaac Newton, Galileo Galilei, Gottfried Wilhelm von Leibnitz, René Descartes, and other giants of physical science, was a period of remarkable progress in the field of physics. It is not surprising then that theorists in the field of medicine, noting the truths discovered by conceiving of nature as a great machine functioning according to laws that could be expressed in mathematical terms, should have attempted to explain the human body as a machine.

William Harvey (1578-1657), whose name looms great in the history of seventeenth-century medicine, explained the circulation of the blood in mechanical terminology. To Harvey, working under the influence of the great physicists, the heart was a mechanical force pump and the blood was analogous to other fluids in motion. How many physicians, practicing in the same intellectual environment as this Englishman, must have carried the mechanical analogy to the extent of thinking of the teeth as scissors, the lungs as bellows, the stomach as a flask, and the viscera as a sieve?

The iatrochemical school existed alongside the iatrophysical. Whereas the iatrophysical thought primarily in terms of matter, forces, and motions, the iatrochemical thought chemical relationships were fundamental. One of the founders of this school, the Dutch scientist Sylvius (1614-72), explained diseases chemically (an approach not completely unlike the humoral of Galen) and treated them on the basis of a supposed chemical reaction between drug and disease. Another leading figure in the iatrochemical school, Thomas Willis (1621-75), was an Englishman. These two advocated the use of drugs at a time when their respective nations were developing great colonial empires rich with the raw materials of pharmacology.

However, it would be an error to think of the medicine of the period, either European or Virginian, only in terms of rational or scientific theories. Treatment was too often based on magic, folklore, and superstition. There were physicians relying upon alchemy and astrology; the Royal Touch was held efficacious; and in the *materia medica* of the period were such substances as foxes' lungs, oils of wolves, and Irish whiskey. Nor should it be forgotten that many of the sick never saw a medical man but relied upon self-treatment.

With theories from the ancient authorities and from experimenting scientists to draw upon, the practicing physicians could deduce therapeutic techniques or justify curative measures, but the emphasis on theory brought with it the danger of ignoring experience and abandoning empirical solutions. Aware that many of his fellow physicians tended to overemphasize theory Thomas Sydenham (1624-89), who received his doctorate of medicine from Cambridge University, recommended personal experience drawn from close observation. He scoffed at physicians who learned medicine in books or laboratory, and never at the bedside. His study of epidemics, his emphasis on geography and climate as casual factors in the genesis of disease, make this Englishman's views and practices especially relevant to the medical history of Virginia where geography and climate did play such important roles in the life of the colony.

The history of surgeons and surgery during the century is less distinguished than that of the physician and his practice. Surgery produced no individuals of the stature and significance of Sydenham nor any revolutionary theories as important as Harvey's. Dissections were made but the knowledge acquired was not applied; amputation was common but not always necessary or effective.

Battle wounds and injuries lay in the province of the surgeon. While the surgeon was primarily concerned with the military, using mechanical force (cutting, tying, setting, and puncturing) in his treatment of body wounds and injuries, physicians on the Continent and in England also filled these functions. For example, physicians in Italy sometimes performed surgical operations they considered worthy of their dignified positions, and in England the licensed physician could practice surgery. On the other hand, surgeons licensed by Oxford University were bound not to practice medicine. Both in France and in England surgeons and barbers held membership in the same guild or corporation, and physicians considered them of inferior social status. The American frontier tended to reduce such professional and social distinctions.

In Europe and England, where medical education was institutionalized to a far greater extent than in colonial Virginia, education explains much of the difference in social status between physician and surgeon. The surgeon learned by apprenticeship to an experienced member of his guild while the physician had to meet certain educational and professional requirements, depending upon local or national law. The best medical education of the period could be had at the great centers of Leyden, Paris, and Montpellier. Cambridge and Oxford also offered a degree in medicine.

Englishmen preferred to study medicine abroad—according to a recent study made by Phyllis Allen and printed in the *Journal of the History of Medicine and Allied Sciences*—because a better education could be obtained there in the same number of years. The Doctorate of Medicine required fourteen years of undergraduate and post-graduate study at Oxford; the Cambridge requirement was similar. Despite reforms during the seventeenth century, education at these universities remained dogmatic and classical. Students usually found their studies dull and their social life stimulating. The more enterprising students could find the new ideas of the period in books not required in their course of study. Cambridge, Oxford, and the Royal College of Physicians all licensed physicians who had survived their education, met certain professional requirements, and passed an examination.

That physicians in England did possess a high social status as well as more extensive formal education is evidenced by a precaution taken by the Virginia Company, to avoid causing displeasure among men of rank, in preparing letters patent. The Company requested of the College of Heralds, in 1609, the setting "in order" of the names of noblemen, knights, and Doctors of Divinity, Law, and Medicine so that their "several worths and degrees" might be recognized when their names were inserted on the patents. Surgeons received no mention.

On the other hand, physicians and surgeons in England might well have come from similar social backgrounds and even on occasions from the same families. When there were three or four sons in the family of a country gentleman, he might have followed the custom of keeping the eldest at home to manage and eventually inherit the estate. The second, then, would be sent to one of the universities in order to follow a profession such as that of physician, lawyer, or clergyman. The third might be apprenticed to an apothecary, surgeon, or a skilled craftsman. This practice should be borne in mind when former medical apprentices are found in high offices in Virginia; their origins were not always humble.

Although the physician enjoyed the greatest social and professional prestige, he received the most verbal abuse and criticism. Perhaps the most damaging and galling satire of the century flowed from the pen of the French dramatist, Molière, who had a medical student—not completely fictitious—swear always to accept the pronouncements of his oldest physician-colleague, and always to treat by purgation, using clysters (enemas), phlebotomy (bloodletting), and emetics (vomitives). These three curative measures followed the best Galenic technique: releasing corrupting humors from the body. Molière's *Le Malade Imaginaire* confronted the audience with constant purgings and bleedings, and the caricature was not excessive.

The diseases of the century did not allow for the inadequacies of the physician, and imparted a grim note of realism to the satire of the dramatist. Infant mortality was high and the life expectancy low. Hardly a household escaped the tragedy of death of the young and the robust; historians have sensed the influence omnipresent death had upon the attitudes and aspirations of the European and American of earlier centuries. School children today learn of such a dramatic killer as the bubonic plague, but even its terrible ravages do not dwarf the toll of ague (malaria), smallpox, typhoid and typhus, diphtheria, respiratory disorders, scurvy, beriberi, and flux (dysentery) in the colonial period.

England, and especially London with its surrounding marshes, suffered acutely with the ague during the century. Englishmen arriving in the New World were well aware of the dangers of this disease and made some effort to avoid the bad air, and the low and damp places. In 1658 the ague took such a toll that a contemporary described the whole island of Britain as a monstrous public hospital. Unfortunately, Thomas Sydenham, whose prestige in England was great and whose works on fevers were influential, paid scant tribute to cinchona bark (quinine) which was known but thought of, even by Sydenham, as only an alleged curative offering too radical a challenge to current techniques. According to humoral doctrine, fever demanded a purging, not the intake of additional substances.

Unfortunately, public hygiene and sanitation enlisted few adherents. Epidemics of the seventeenth century have been judged the most severe in history. In Italy physicians ahead of their times proposed the draining of marshes and pools of stagnant water, and recommended the isolation of persons with contagious diseases. But it was the great London fire of 1666 that rid that city of its infested and infected places, not an enlightened municipality.

Therefore Virginia, a colony of seventeenth-century Europe, started life burdened with a heritage of deadly and widespread disease and inadequate medicine. Not only did the ships that brought the settlers to Jamestown Island bring surgeons and medical supplies but also medical problems frequently more serious than the men and supplies could cope with.

The European or Englishman, however, did not originate the practice of medicine in Virginia for the Indian had had to struggle with the problems of disease and injury long before the seventeenth century.

INDIANS AND THEIR MEDICINE

Seventeenth-century Americans found the medical practices of the Indians interesting enough to include descriptions of them in their accounts of the New World. The attitude of the authors of these early observations is a mixture of curiosity, wonder, and—on occasion—admiration.

Henry Spelman, one of the early colonists, wrote of Jamestown and Virginia as they were in 1609 and 1610. He described the manner of visiting with the sick among the Indians. According to Spelman, the "preest" laid the sick Indian upon a mat and, sitting down beside him, placed a bowl of water and a rattle between them. Taking the water into his mouth and spraying it over the Indian, the priest then began to beat his chest and make noises with the rattle. Rising, he shook the rattle over all of his patient's body, rubbed the distressed parts with his hands, and then sprinkled water over him again.

Like the colonist, the Indian tried to draw out blood or other matter from the sick or wounded person. The method often used for releasing the ill humor from a painful joint or limb must have caused considerable suffering but may have offered certain advantages in preventing fatal infection. If the affected part could bear it, the Indian thrust a smoldering pointed stick deep into the sore place and kept it there until the excess matter could drain off. Another technique for burning and opening had a small cone of slowly burning wood inserted in the distressed place, "letting it burn out upon the part, which makes a running sore effectually."

Still another method for treating a wound was for the priest to gash open the wound with a small bit of flint, suck the blood and other matter from it, and finally apply to it the powder of a root. A colonist in describing the practice wrote that "they have many professed phisitions, who with their charmes and rattels, with an infernall rowt of words and actions, will seeme to sucke their inwarde griefe from their navels or their grieved places." Judging by other accounts written during the century concerning Indian medicine, the powdered root may well have been sassafras, of which there was an abundance in the Jamestown area. The priest dried the root in the embers of a fire, scraped off the outer bark, powdered it, and bound the wound after applying the powder.

Not only did the native American resort to a crude form of bloodletting but he practiced sweating as well—which was also common to seventeenth-century European medical practice. In Captain John Smith's description of Virginia it was noted that when troubled with "dropsies, swellings, aches, and such like diseases" the cure was to build a stove "in the form of a dovehouse with mats, so close that a fewe coales therein covered with a pot, will make the pacient sweate extremely."

Before lighting his stove, the Indian covered his sweating place with bark so close that no air could enter. When he began to sweat profusely, the sick Indian dashed out from his heated shelter and into a nearby creek, sea, or river. An Englishman commented that after returning to his hut again he "either recover[s] or give[s] up the ghost."

The Indians, like Molière's stage physician, believed in the value of the purge. Every spring they deliberately made themselves sick with drinking the juices of a medicinal root. The dosage purged them so thoroughly that they did not recover until three or four days later. The Indians also ate green corn in the spring to work the same effect.

The Indian medicine man, like his European counterpart, frequently dispensed medicines or drugs. As has been the custom among many men in the medical profession, the medicine man would not reveal the secrets of his medicines. "Made very knowing in the hidden qualities of plants and other natural things," he considered it a part of the obligations of his priesthood to conceal the information from all but those who were to succeed him. On the other hand, the Indian priest showed his concern for the health of his people—and the similarity of his attitude to that of present day practices— by making an exception to his canon of secrecy in the case of drugs needed in emergencies arising on a hunting trip and during travel.

According to one early eighteenth-century history of Virginia, the Indian in choosing raw materials for drugs preferred roots and barks of trees to the leaves of plants or trees. If the drug were to be taken internally it was mixed with water; when juices were to be applied externally they were left natural unless water was necessary for moistening. Whatever the drug and however utilized, the Indian called it *wisoccan* or *wighsacan*, for this term was not a specific herb, as some of the earlier settlers thought, but a general term.

Besides sassafras, medicinal roots and barks, the Indian believed in beneficial effects of a kind of clay called *wapeig*. The clay, in the opinion of the Indians, cured sores and wounds; an English settler marvelled to find in use "a strange kind of earth, the vertue whereof I know not; but the Indians eate it for physicke, alleaging that it cureth the sicknesse and paine of the belly." Insomuch as the Indian priest preferred to keep his professional secrets, the colonist was unlikely ever to learn the "vertue" of the clay.

If the Indian medicine man had not believed that his gods would be displeased—or his prestige lowered—by revealing the nature of the *wisoccan* he prescribed, it would have been possible for the early Virginians to have drawn upon the Indian knowledge of, and experience with, the simples and therapies of the New World. (Perhaps the "vertues" of the clay would have cured the "paines" of the Jamestown bellies.) As it was, the settlers make little mention of a reliance upon the Indians for medical assistance.

CHAPTER TWO

Disease and The Critical Years At Jamestown

MOTIVES AND PROVISIONS FOR COLONIZATION

In 1606 King James of England granted a charter to Sir Thomas Gates and others authorizing settlements in the New World. In 1609 this charter was revised and enlarged, granting the privileges to a joint-stock company. Among the merchants, knights, and gentlemen holding shares in the company and among those particularly interested in the more southerly areas of North America, including Virginia, were a number of physicians. The instructions given to the first settlers reflect the general concern of the London Company for the health of the colony and perhaps the particular interest of the physicians. One of the physicians, John Woodall, took especial care to urge that cattle be sent to provide the settlers with the milk he considered essential to their health.

Not only did the Company wish to lessen the dangers of disease in the New World, but it also urged colonization as a means of reducing the plague in England. In 1609 the Company advised municipal authorities in London to remove the excess population of that great city to Virginia as the surplus was thought to be a cause of the plague. There was little danger of a surplus population during the initial years in Virginia.

Before the colonists, or the Company, however, had to be concerned with dangers from disease in Virginia, the colonists had to undertake an extremely difficult and unhealthy voyage across the Atlantic.

DISEASE AND THE OCEAN VOYAGE

Ships plying the Atlantic at the beginning of the seventeenth century were small and the voyage was lengthy. Four months passed before the *Godspeed*, the *Discovery*, and the *Susan Constant*, carrying the first permanent settlers to Jamestown, sighted the two capes at the mouth of Chesapeake Bay in April, 1607.

Although these small ships carrying the first permanent settlers had a stopover in the West Indies for rest and replenishment, there had been debilitating months at sea and more than 100 emigrants to provide for in addition to the crews. With limited cargo and passenger space, water and food supplies could hardly satisfy the demand created by a hundred persons at sea for hundreds of days. Several of the emigrants died on the first voyage and the remainder disembarked poorly prepared for the new tests their constitutions would soon endure.

The sea voyage of these first settlers probably exacted no heavier a death toll and caused no more suffering because the ships went by way of the Canaries and the West Indies instead of by the more northerly route by-passing the islands. A contemporary described the advantages thought to be had from the stopover in the West Indies (at the island of Nevis):

We came to a bath standing in a valley betwixt two hills, where wee bathed ourselves.... Finding this place to be so convenient for our men to avoid diseases which will breed in so long a voyage, wee incamped our selves on this ile six dayes, and spent none of our ships victuall.

Anchoring off other West Indian islands the ships were able to replenish their stores with fresh meat and fish and to replace the evil-smelling and foul water in their casks with fresh. By these measures the colonists demonstrated a concern not only for comfort but also for hygienic precautions.

Later voyages during the century took anywhere from two to three months. Despite the precautions taken by some, of a rest, in the West Indies to bring about "restitution of our sick people into health by the helpes of fresh ayre, diet and the baths," the trip aboard the pestered ships continued to exact a heavy death toll and to discharge disease and diseased persons. Benefits resulting from the stopover in the Indies were countered by the considerable exposure to tropical infections. One convoy carrying colonists to Virginia in 1609 and running a southerly course through "fervent heat and loomes breezes" had many of the crew and passengers fall ill from calenture (tropical or yellow fever). Out of two ships so afflicted, thirty-two persons died and were thrown overboard. Another of these ships reported the plague raging in her.

Irritated by frequent references to the unhealthy climate of Virginia and fearful that the bad publicity would increase the difficulties in obtaining colonists, officials of the London Company took pains to expose the part that the ocean voyage played in bringing about the deaths of newcomers. Musty bread and stinking beer aboard the pestered ships, according to a contemporary, worked as a chief cause of the mortality attributed falsely to the Virginia climate and conditions at Jamestown. In 1624 Governor Wyatt and his associates recommended to commissioners from England that "care must be had that the ships come not over pestered and that they may be well used at sea with that plenty and goodness of dyet as is promised in England but seldom performed." Others complained of the crowding of men in their own "aires," uncleanliness of the ships, and the presence of fatal "infexion."

Insomuch as seventeenth-century medical theory paid scant attention to sanitation and hygiene in the study of the causes of disease, it is surprising to find the early Virginian rightly recognizing the ships as sources of sickness. On the other hand, observation could not help but lead passengers to conclude that sickness, such as flux or dysentery, with which they had to suffer aboard ship, might have a causal relationship to the ship. To have related the transmission of the plague from epidemic centers in England via infected shipboard rats, and transmission of tropical fevers, as well, by the medium of shipboard water buckets infected with mosquito larvae from the tropics, was beyond the capacity of both medical theory and of first-hand observation.

Physicians or surgeons did ship aboard the seventeenth-century ocean-going vessels, but Doctor Wyndham B. Blanton, the chief authority on seventeenth-century Virginia medicine, concludes that most of them probably had poor educations and little more to recommend them than "a smattering of drugs, a little practice in opening abscesses and a liking for the sea." A seventeenth-century contemporary recommended that a ship's surgeon—surgeons went to sea far more often than physicians—be the possessor of a certificate from a barber-surgeon guild and be freed from all ship's duties except the attending of the sick and the cure of the wounded. The ship's surgeon, then, crossed the professional line between surgeon and physician, a line that necessity would soon force so many medical men to cross in America.

Throughout the century ship's surgeons abandoned their shipboard duties to settle in the Virginia colony, and there seems little reason to doubt that those remaining aboard ship took advantage of the opportunity when in port to help meet the medical needs of the colonists, thus supplementing the medical talent which had taken up residence in Virginia.

The labors of the ship's surgeon at sea, no matter how valiant, could not offset the miseries of the long sea voyage, and the sight of Virginia's coast greatly cheered all hands. After the foul air, crowded quarters, and inadequate provisions of the ship, many settlers must have reacted to the Virginia land as Captain John Smith did: "heaven and earth never agree better to frame a place for man's habitation." It is not surprising then that the first permanent settlers were somewhat less than careful when evaluating, against standards of health, the possible sites for settlement.

THE SELECTION OF SITES FOR SETTLEMENT

In a fairly extensive set of instructions "by way of advice, for the intended voyage to Virginia," the London Company, in 1606, took into account the part that disease and famine could play in the life—or death—of the colony. Probably knowing that the chances for survival of the Spanish conquistadors had been enhanced by their superhuman qualities in the eyes of the Indians, the Company urged that no information on deaths or sicknesses among the whites be allowed to the natives. More important, as the course of events was to demonstrate, was the advice not to:

plant in a low or moist place, because it will prove unhealthfull. You shall judge of the good air by the people; for some part of that coast where the lands are low, have their people blear eyed, and with swollen bellies and legs: but if the naturals be strong and clean made, it is a true sign of wholesome soil.

The idea that climate had an influence upon human physiognomy did not originate with the London Company. In an essay dating back to the fifth century B.C. and preserved among the works of the Hippocratic school the ancient—but in the seventeenth century still influential—authorities argued that human physiognomies could be classified into the well-wooded and well-watered mountain type; the thin-soiled waterless type; the well-cleared and well-drained lowland type; and the meadowy, marshy type.

The London Company's instructions to the first permanent settlers to avoid low-lying, marshy land, if followed, might have saved the colonists from some of the sicknesses they were to endure, but other considerations dictated the choice of the Jamestown site; the peninsular, about thirty miles upstream, provided natural protection and a good view up and down the river. The danger from the ships of other European peoples seemed more immediate and formidable than those from the mosquito, with its breeding place in the nearby swamp, and from the foul and brackish drinking water.

As the century progressed, the settlers pushed inland from Jamestown and the low-lying coastal region, up onto the drier land. The danger from typhoid, dysentery, and malaria grew steadily less. In choosing home sites—once the confines of the peninsula were left behind and the fear of attack from Indian or European was less—the early planters took into consideration the dangers of the fetid swamp and muggy lowland.

That the promotion of health did play a part in the selection of sites for settlement is borne out by the re-location of the seat of government from the languishing village of Jamestown to Middle Plantation or Williamsburg. After an accidental fire destroyed a large part of Jamestown at the end of the century, the people indicated a desire to move away from an environment, recognized as unhealthful, to Middle Plantation, known for its temperate, healthy climate as well as for its wholesome springs. The inhabitants had contemplated a move earlier in the century for health reasons but authorities in England and governors in Virginia acted to prevent the abandonment of the only community even approaching the status of a town.

The move away from Jamestown would probably appear a wise measure even to the twentieth-century physician; to the seventeenth-century physician, who often saw a close relationship between climatic conditions and disease, the move seemed imperative. A man well-versed in science and medicine, living in Jamestown a decade or so before the town was abandoned, exemplified this medical theory when he wrote that an area was unhealthy according to its nearness to salt water. He had observed that salt air, especially when stagnant, had "fatal effects" on human bodies. In contrast, clear air (such as would be enjoyed at Middle Plantation) had beneficial effects.

Considerations of health and the effects of disease not only influenced the settlers in their choice of living sites but also in many of their other activities. Political, economic, and social history in seventeenth-century Virginia was determined in part by health and disease.

DISEASE AS A DETERMINING FACTOR IN THE EARLY YEARS OF THE COLONY

Death from disease and incapacitation from disease are challenges to which every civilization—and human community—must successfully respond in order to survive. Historian Arnold J. Toynbee has emphasized the vital character of the challenge and response relationship in the history of all communities. A particular challenge to which early Jamestown almost succumbed was disease. The actions—or inactions—of the settlers under the London Company, 1607-1624, demonstrated especially well the influence of the challenge of disease upon the early history of Virginia.

During the first year of the settlement at Jamestown, disease worked as an important factor in the realm of politics. In this connection, Edward Maria Wingfield, chosen first president of the governing council in Virginia, found himself removed from office, imprisoned, and sent home by the spring of 1608, all as a result of charges brought against him that for the most part were petty and contradictory. Pettiness and contradictions, in this instance, were rooted in the miserable conditions which the colonists had to endure their first summer: famine and sickness not only demoralized the colonists but were killing them faster than they could be buried.

Wingfield left office as president of the council after the first summer spent in Jamestown. The sickness that caused much tension during his tenure was probably the malady loosely described by early Virginians as the "seasoning." The complex of symptoms ascribed to the seasoning bothered the settlers throughout the seventeenth century. Even as late as 1723 a recent arrival in Virginia wrote that "all that come to this country have ordinarily sickness at first which they call a seasoning of which I shall assure you I had a most severe one." During the first two summers, 1607 and 1608, however, this seasoning inflicted the most distress, judging by the seriousness with which contemporaries described it.

One of these contemporary accounts, written by George Percy who sailed to Virginia with the first settlers in 1606-07, described the distress caused by seasoning and famine during the summer of 1607. The awfulness of that summer is made more dramatic by the manner in which Percy introduced the subject. Having described the voyage over, which was relatively pleasant with the stopover in the beautiful West Indian islands, and having entertained the reader with startling accounts of the habits of the savages in Virginia ("making many devillish gestures with a hellish noise, foming at the mouth, staring with their eyes, wagging their heads and hands in such a fashion and deformitie as it was monstrous to behold"), Percy abruptly began listing the names of the dead as his narrative moved into the late summer months:

The sixt of August there died John Asbie of the bloudie flixe. The ninth day died George Flowre of the swelling.... The fifteenth day, their died Edward Browne and Stephen Galthorpe. The sixteenth day, their died Thomas Gower Gentleman. The seventeenth day, their died Thomas Mounslic....

The remainder of the description of the significant events of the month of August is given over entirely to the listing of the deaths. Seldom did Percy give the cause of individual deaths, but as the narrative moved into September and near the end of the seasoning period, Percy stopped his grim listing to comment in general terms upon the unhappy experience.

According to his diagnosis—and perhaps he was enlightened by Thomas Wotton and Will Wilkinson, the two surgeons who arrived with the first settlers—the heavy death toll of August resulted from such ailments as fluxes, swellings, and burning fevers as well as from famine and attacks by the Indians.

Percy was of the opinion that the colonists at Jamestown suffered more during the summer and winter of 1607 than any other Englishmen have during a colonization venture. Weakened by the debilitating summer and unable during that period to make the necessary provisions for the winter, the settlers, their ranks depleted, also fared poorly during the next five months.

In describing their distress, he revealed the conditions that bred the diseases and illnesses to which the colonists fell prey. They lay on the bare ground through weather cold and hot, dry and wet, and their ration of food consisted of a small can of barley sod in water—one can for five men. Drinking water came from the river which in turn was salt at high tide, and slimy and filthy at low. With such food and drink, the small contingent within the fort lay about for weeks "night and day groaning in every corner ... most pittifull to heare."

Fortunately during the course of the winter the Indians did come to the relief of the colonists with provisions, but before this help was substantial, Percy observed:

If there were any conscience in men, it would make their harts to bleed to heare the pitifull murmurings and out-cries of our sick men without reliefe, every night and day, for the space of sixe weekes, some departing out the world, many times three or foure in a night; in the morning, their bodies trailed out of their cabines like dogges to be buried.

Over one-half (approximately 60) of the original settlers perished during the summer of 1607 and the seasoning was to prove a hazard throughout the remainder of the century. Its effects became less serious, however, as the Company and the colonists, profiting from the earlier experiences began to plan departures from England so that the immigrants would arrive in Virginia in the fall: another example of the influence of disease.

Governor Yeardley, writing some years later—in 1620—reminded the Company's officials in England of the advantages of a fall arrival. He had just witnessed the distress of immigrants from three ships that had arrived in May:

had they arrived at a seasonable time of the year I would not have doubted of their lives and healths, but this season is most unfit for people to arrive here ... some [came] very weak and sick, some crazy and tainted ashore, and now this great heat of weather striketh many more but for life.

At least twenty more immigrants died during the second summer (1608) and the misery and discontent of the survivors of the summer's sicknesses account—in part, at least—for the disposal of another council president, John Ratcliffe. Returning to Jamestown after an exploratory trip up Chesapeake Bay, Doctor Walter Russell, one of the company, found the latest arrivals to Virginia "al sicke, the rest, some lame, some bruised, al unable to do any thing but complain of the pride and unreasonable needlesse cruelty of their sillie President." The wrath of these sick—and doubtless somewhat querulous and irrational men—was appeased by the removal of the "sillie" president.

The ability of Captain John Smith, who succeeded to the presidency of the council in the fall of 1608, to impose his strong will upon the inhabitants of the peninsula, and to exert such a great influence upon the course of events is explained, in part, by the depletion of ranks and the demoralization of spirit caused among them by the dreadful toll of disease. When other members of the council died, Smith did not replace them and, rid of strong opposition, he ruled as a benevolent despot.

Smith's departure from the colony in October, 1609, had as its immediate cause—according to Smith—the impossibility of his obtaining proper medical attention in Virginia for burns acquired from a gunpowder explosion. When Smith sailed, his enemies, of which there were a considerable number, breathed freer air, but the colony subsequently suffered without his strong, authoritative voice.

Supporters of Smith argued that if that "unhappy" accident had not occurred, he could have stayed on and solved the many problems that were to beset the colony. On the other hand, it is pointed out that the wound would have been better treated at Jamestown than on board ship, and that Smith used the wound, which was not too serious, as an excuse to escape from the administrative troubles that plagued him.

The powder blast was described by friends of Smith as tearing a nine or ten-inch square of flesh from his body and thighs, and as causing him such torment that he could not carry out the duties of his position. The wound was probably complicated by the fact that the accident had occurred when Smith was in a boat many miles from Jamestown. He had had to cover the great return distance after having plunged into the water to ease his agony, and without having the assistance of either medicines or medical treatment. Whatever the seriousness of the wound, supporters of Smith maintained that he was near death and had to leave Jamestown in order to secure the services of "chirurgian and chirurgery... [to] cure his hurt."

Twice in 1608, Captain Newport had brought immigrants and supplies to the colony and, in the summer of 1609 about 400 passengers had landed at Jamestown. These new arrivals, some of them already afflicted with the plague, others victims of various fevers, and all suffering from malnutrition, needed strong leadership to force them to plant busily and to lay in food supplies for the winter ahead. Supplies brought over aboard the ships could not possibly furnish nourishment for the coming months. Malnutrition as a factor contributing to sickness, and sickness as a factor preventing the labor necessary to circumvent starvation, constituted a vicious relationship.

The winter of 1609-10 after Smith's departure is remembered as the "Starving Time." During this period the number of colonists dropped from 500 to about sixty. Men, women, and children lived—or died—eating roots, herbs, acorns, walnuts, berries, and an occasional fish. They ate horses, dogs, mice, and snakes without hesitation after Indians drove off hogs and deer belonging to the colonists. The Indians also kept the settlers from leaving the protection of Jamestown to go out and hunt for food. When hunting was not made impossible by Indians, the settlers' own physical weaknesses often precluded energetic action.

The notorious, and possibly untrue, incident of the man whom hunger drove to kill and to eat the salted remains of his wife, is from the accounts of the Starving Time. Although this story had the support of a number of colonists, others maintain that it, and the entire episode of the famine, came out of the exaggeration of colonists who abandoned the venture and returned to England. Yet the verdict of historians establishes a Starving Time, and the high mortality of the winter must have an explanation.

To argue that all those who died, died of starvation would, on the other hand, be a distortion. Food deficiencies did not always lead directly to death but in many cases to dietary disease. These dietary diseases often terminated in death, but their courses might well not have been fatal if proper medical attention could have been given. In other cases food deficiency resulted in so weakened a physical condition that the body fell prey to infectious diseases which, again, could not be cured with the limited medical help available.

The Starving Time did not stand out as a time of want to be contrasted with a normal time of plenty. For many the winter of 1609-10 only brought to a crisis dietary disorders of long standing. One account of the early years describes the daily ration as eight ounces of meal and a half-pint of peas, both "the one and the other being mouldy, rotten, full of cobwebs and maggots loathsome to man and not fytt for beasts...."

Nor was the Starving Time the last time that the colonists would have to endure famine and privation. Although written to discredit the administration of Sir Thomas Smith as head of the Company during the years from 1607-19, an account of the hunger of these twelve years should be accepted as having some basis in fact. The account, written in 1624, reported as common occurrences the stealing of food by the starving and the cruel punishments meted out to them (one for "steelinge of 2 or 3 pints of oatemeal had a bodkinge thrust through his tounge and was tyed with a chaine to a tree untill he starved"); and the denial of an allowance of food to men who were too sick to work ("soe consequently perished").

The starving colonists during these twelve years, according to the report, often resorted to dogs, cats, rats, snakes, horsehides, and other extremes for nourishment. Many, in those hungry times, weary of life, dug holes in the earth and remained there hidden from the authorities until dead from starvation. Although the report maintained that these events occurred throughout the twelve-year period, it is likely that many were concentrated during the Starving Time.

Famished, disease-ridden, demoralized, with many mentally unbalanced, the settlement at Jamestown languished in a distressful condition after the winter of 1609-10. Jamestown, in May, 1610 appeared:

as the ruins of some auntient [for]tification then that any people living might now inhabit it: the pallisadoes... tourne downe, the portes open, the gates from the hinges, the church ruined and unfrequented, empty howses (whose owners untimely death had taken newly from them) rent up and burnt, the living not hable, as they pretended, to step into the woodes to gather other fire-wood; and, it is true, the *Indian as fast killing without as the famine and pestilence within.*

The Indians, however, would not make a direct assault on the fort; they waited on disease and famine to destroy the remaining whites. How many of the graves now at Jamestown must have been dug during that terrible winter? The Starving Time has been characterized by historian Oliver Chitwood as "the most tragic experience endured by any group of pioneers who had a part in laying the foundations of the present United States."

By spring of 1610 the challenge of famine, pestilence, and disease had proven too great; the warfare of Europeans and savages, for which the settlers had made provisions in the selection of the Jamestown site, had not proven as great a threat as disease and famine. Under the command of Sir Thomas Gates and Sir George Somers, who had only just arrived with plans for the future of the settlement, the small band of survivors boarded ship to abandon an abortive experiment in European colonization.

Before leaving, the survivors of the winter had had a consultation with Gates and Somers about future prospects for the colony. Chiefly fear of starvation determined the decision to abandon the settlement: the provisions brought by Gates and Somers would have lasted only sixteen days. The colonists could hold out no hope of obtaining food from the Indians. ("It soone then appeared most fitt, by general approbation, that to preserve and save all from starving, there could be no readier course thought on then to abandon the countrie.")

After embarking, the settlers, with Gates, Somers, and the new arrivals, had reached the mouth of the river when they met Lord De la Warr, the new governor of the colony, coming from England with fresh supplies and settlers. Heartened, the survivors of the Starving Time turned back to try the New World again.

In Lord De la Warr's company was Dr. Lawrence Bohun, a physician of good reputation, who subsequently distinguished himself serving the medical needs of the settlement. He could not, however, even in his capacity of personal physician, prevent Lord De la Warr from falling victim to the common ailments.

In 1610, Lord De la Warr wrote: "presently after my arrival in Jamestowne, I was welcomed by a hot and violent ague, which held mee a time, till by the advice of my physician, Doctor Lawrence Bohun I was recovered." Bohun, in the seventeenth-century tradition of treatment by clysters, vomitives, and phlebotomy, resorted to bloodletting. The letting, believed to free the body of fermented blood and malignant humors, probably gave the governor a psychological lift, if only a temporary one.

De la Warr, who blamed the distress of the colony upon the failures of the settlers, soon had another taste of the illnesses which so many of the colonists endured during their first months in the New World. In his report to the Company explaining his early departure from the colony, he included one of the fullest surviving accounts of sickness at Jamestown during the first few years of settlement:

That disease [the hot and violent ague] had not long left me, til (within three weekes after I had gotten a little strength) I began to be distempered with other greevous sicknesses, which successively and severally assailed me: for besides a relapse into the former disease, which with much more violence held me more than a moneth, and brought me to great weakenesse, the flux surprised me, and kept me many daies: then the crampe assaulted my weak body, with strong paines; and afterwards the gout (with which I had heeretofore beene sometime troubled) afflicted mee in such sort, that making my body through weakenesse unable to stirre, or to use any maner of exercies, drew upon me the disease called the scurvy; which though in others it be a sicknesse of slothfulnesse, yet was in me an effect of weaknesse, which never left me, till I was upon the point to leave the world.

When a person of strong constitution, living under the best conditions the colony could provide, and accompanied by a well-trained physician, found himself thus incapacitated, it is no wonder that the rank and file of the colony failed to pursue energetically by hard work and exemplary conduct their own best interests.

The firmness of De la Warr, who was much more indulgent of his own than of others' disorders, brought additional stability to the colony, but the attack of scurvy, which current opinion believed could be relieved only by the citrous fruits of the West Indies, caused him, accompanied by Dr. Bohun, to set sail from Virginia in the spring of 1611 for the same island of Nevis praised so highly for its baths by the first settlers of 1607. Disease had robbed the colony of another outstanding leader during a period when strong leadership on the scene was imperative.

Although the colony had experienced its worst years of hardship before De la Warr departed and the worst years in the New World had been caused by famine and disease, sickness and starvation were still to have a noteworthy effect. Disease no longer threatened the colony's life, but it shaped its history.

In 1624 the charter of the Company was annulled and, in explaining this major development, account must be taken of the cumulative effects of sickness and hunger upon the Company's fortunes; the first summer's seasoning and the Starving Time, for example, had long-term economic repercussions as well as short-term results in human suffering.

The Company had been in financial difficulties for some years and by 1624 the treasury was empty and the indebtedness heavy. If the mortality rate had not been so high and the level of energy of the colonists so reduced, the Company might have prospered. For example, local trade with the Indians necessitated small ships for the effective transportation of cargo, but several attempts by the Company to send to America boatwrights to construct such ships failed because of the deaths of the boatwrights. The Company had hoped in 1620 to better its financial condition by developing an iron industry in the colony, but this project suffered from the effects of disease, too, as the chief men for the iron works died during the ocean voyage. The remainder of the officers and men sent to establish the works died in Virginia either from disease or at the hands of the Indians. The high cost to the Company of the labor and services lost because of the early deaths of persons still indentured for a period of years cannot be estimated. Nor can the number of goals set by the colonists and the Company but never fulfilled because of sickness be tabulated. As late as 1623 a colonist wrote that "these slow supplies, which hardly rebuild every year the decays of the former, retain us only in a languishing state and curb us from the carrying of enterprise of moment."

In suggesting the part that famine and disease played in the annulment of the Company's charter, the effects of one more period of intense suffering must also be considered. In March, 1622, a bloody Indian massacre occurred in which more than 350 white men, women, and children died. Not only did the massacre cause a subsequent period of disease, famine, and death among the survivors, but the heavy casualties inflicted directly by the Indians can be explained, partially, by the weakened condition and depleted ranks of the colonists before the massacre.

So tenuous was the colony's ability to maintain an adequate and healthful living standard, that the destructive and disrupting impact of the massacre brought a period of severe famine and sickness. After the raid the surviving colonists had to abandon many of the outlying plantations with their arable fields, livestock, and supplies. And having had the routine of life interrupted, the settlers—their numbers unfortunately increased by a large supply of new immigrants, sent by ambitious planners in England—came to the winter of 1622-23 poorly provisioned.

Toward the end of this winter, famine reduced the settlers to such conditions that one wrote to his parents that he had often eaten more at home in a day than in Virginia in a week. The beggar in England without his limbs seemed fortunate to the Virginian who had to live day after day on a scant ration of peas, water-gruel, and a small portion of bread. Another wrote that the settlers died like rotten sheep and "full of maggots as he can hold. They rot above ground." As in 1609-10, inadequate diet weakened the body and made it easy prey to infection.

During this winter the colonists—in addition to suffering from want of food—had to endure a "pestilent fever" of epidemic proportions matched only by the seasoning of 1607. About 500 persons died in the course of the winter.

The origin of the winter's epidemic, according to contemporaries, lay in the infectious conditions of numbers of the immigrants who had been poisoned during the ocean voyage "with stinking beer" supplied to the ships by Mr. Dupper of London. It is more likely that the pestilent fever of the winter was a respiratory disease rather than a disorder resulting from "stinking beer." Another commentator on the winter called attention to the continued "wadinge and wettinge" the colonists had to endure, bringing them cold upon cold until "they leave to live."

Whether continual wadings and wettings brought on respiratory diseases, or bad beer dietary, is debatable, but the critics of the Company used the dreadful winter of 1622-23 to discredit its administration. They pointed out that the Company had sent large numbers of immigrants to Virginia without proper provisions, and to a colony without adequate means of providing food and shelter for them. Many of these persons had subsequently died during the winter of 1622-23.

The Company, embarrassed by failures in Virginia—many of which resulted directly from unhappy combinations of famine and disease—and plagued by political dissension and economic difficulties, had its charter annulled in May, 1624. One of the most adversely critical—and somewhat prejudiced—tracts written against the Company summed up conditions in the colony after fifteen years under its direction:

There havinge been as it is thought not fewer than tenn thousand soules transported thither ther are not through the aforenamed abuses and neglects above two thousand of them at the present to be found alive, many of them alsoe in a sickly and desperate estate. Soe that itt may undoubtedly [be expected that unless the defects of administration be remedied] that in steed of a plantacion it will shortly gett the name of a slaughterhouse....

The Company did not live on after 1624 to acquire such a name, but during its short—and unhealthy—existence the effects of disease on history were manifest. Company instructions gave attention to health requirements; ocean sailings depended upon health conditions; famine and disease almost caused the early abandonment of the colony; strong administrators left, for reasons of health, a Virginia sorely in need of leadership; poor health conditions resulting in lowered morale undermined local leaders; and the over-all economic welfare of the colony suffered from the long-term and short-term effects of famine and disease. The intimate or personal hardships endured by the individual settlers because of disease and famine cannot be enumerated, but the persistent influence that the summation of all the individual suffering had on the general spirit and ethics of early Virginia cannot be overlooked.

Disease and famine did not cease to influence Virginia history in 1624, but their great importance during the first two decades has been emphasized because they were then a factor exerting a major influence, perhaps the predominant one.

CHAPTER THREE

Prevalent Ills and Common Treatments

COMMON AND UNCOMMON DISEASES

As has been noted, the seasoning caused great distress and a high mortality among the new arrivals to the colony throughout the seventeenth century. These Virginians—authorities on medicine or not—had, for the origins of this malady, their own explanations which furnish clues for more recent analysis. The general term "seasoning" is of little assistance to the medical historian attempting to understand three hundred year-old illnesses in twentieth-century terms.

According to seventeenth-century contemporaries, the pathology of seasoning might be described as follows. The immigrants disembarked from their ships tired and underfed—generally in poor health. From their ships they took up residence in a Jamestown without adequate food supplies of its own, and without shelter for the new arrivals. Many of the new settlers had to sleep outside, regardless of the weather, for a number of days after arrival. Then they exposed themselves to the burning rays of the sun, the "gross and vaporous aire and soyle" of Jamestown, and drank its foul and brackish water.

The foul and brackish drinking water would seem to be the most probable casual agent in the opinion of more recent medical authority. In this water, Dr. Blanton believes, lurked the deadly typhoid bacillus—the killer behind the mask of the seasoning. Typhoid is not the only possibility, but burning fever, the flux (diarrhea), and the bellyache—symptoms listed in the early accounts—indicate typhoid. Other diseases that may have caused the seasoning were dysentery, influenza, and malaria; and these may have been the seasoning during some of the later summers of the century.

Whatever diseases may have caused the seasoning, it plagued the colony summer after summer. A Dutch ship captain wrote of it as it was in Virginia in the summer of 1633:

There is an objection which the English make. They say that during the months of June, July, and August it is very unhealthy; that their people, who have then lately arrived from England, die during these months like cats and dogs, ... when they have the sickness, they want to sleep all the time, but they must be prevented from sleeping by force, as they die if they get asleep.

Sir Francis Wyatt, twice governor of Virginia wrote, "but certaine it is new comers seldome passe July and August without a burning fever—this requires a skilful phisitian, convenient diett and lodging with diligent attendance." The skillful physician could not limit himself, however, to the curing of the seasoning; he had many other maladies in Virginia with which to contend: dietary disorders, malaria, plague, yellow fever, smallpox, respiratory disorders, and a host of other diseases.

Beriberi and scurvy, both dietary diseases, handicapped the colony throughout the century, and probably had acute manifestations during the Starving Time of 1609-10. The colonists during the early years at Jamestown often boiled their limited rations in a common kettle, thus destroying what little valuable vitamin content the food may have had; eggs, vegetables, and fruits which would have countered the disease were not available. The swellings and the deaths without obvious cause described by the early commentators may have resulted from beriberi (the disease did not have a name until the eighteenth century).

Another dietary disease troubling the colonists but, unlike beriberi, known by name and at times properly treated, was scurvy. Mention has been made of the outbreak of this disease aboard the ships, and of the stops made in the West Indies to eat the health-restoring citrus fruits, but in the case of the colonists at Jamestown the fruit was non-existent. A belief, also held, that idleness caused the disease did little to bring about measures to promote proper treatment. Because the incapacitating aspects of the disease could produce the appearance of idleness, numerous ill persons must have been innocently stigmatized. Their situation became hopeless when denied rations because the authorities wished to discipline the apparently lazy.

Insomuch as the ague (or malaria) exacted a high toll in seventeenth-century Europe—especially in England—it would be reasonable to assume that, with typhoid and dietary disorders, this disease caused most of the illness in Virginia. When emphasis has been placed, by authorities, upon the location of Jamestown as a disease-producing factor, the implication has often been that the swampy area was a mosquito and malaria breeding place. A number of historians have asserted that malaria produced the highest mortality figures at Jamestown. Much is also made of the tragic circumstance that the arresting agent for the disease, cinchona bark or quinine, was known on the European continent by mid-seventeenth century but that little use was made of it.

Dr. Blanton, the authority on seventeenth-century Virginia medicine, in contrast argues that "there is not evidence ... that malaria was responsible for a preponderating part of the great mortalities of the Seventeenth Century in Virginia." He bases this conclusion on a number of facts: he has been able to find only five or six references to the ague (malaria) in the records of the century; because the ague was well-known he does not believe its symptoms, such as the racking chill, would have escaped notice. On the other hand, he does not doubt the presence of the ague in Virginia throughout the century even though it did not cause the most distress.

As in the case of the ague, a reasonable assumption would be that the plague existed in seventeenth-century Virginia. The Great Plague of London (1665) carried away 69,000 persons, and other cities of Europe had even more disastrous epidemics. During the two years before the first settlers arrived at Jamestown, over 2000 victims were buried in London. The accounts of the ocean voyage indicate rat-infested ships. Ships of the London Company reported plague and death aboard. Virginians took pains to describe their illnesses, and there would have been little difficulty in recognizing this well-known killer. Yet little evidence of the presence of the plague appears in the seventeenth-century Virginia record; cases are reported but the number is small. Why Virginia should have been spared—especially in view of the known rat-infestation aboard ship—remains a question.

The evidence relative to yellow fever, or calenture, during this period in Virginia is contradictory. Early sources do make reference to numerous deaths from it at sea and even to an epidemic of it at Jamestown before 1610, but subsequent notices are infrequent and of questionable validity. Prevalence of the disease in the earlier years and its comparative infrequency in later is not a likely circumstance because with the increase of commerce, especially from tropical ports, an increase of the disease should have followed.

Smallpox, the mark of which is seen in early portraits, emerges from the colonial record with a more reasonable history. Its incidence in Virginia during the first half of the seventeenth century was small, and this might be expected in view of the fact that there were few children in the colony and that most of the adults had been infected before they left the Old World. The number of smallpox epidemics in Virginia did increase—again, as might be expected—later in the century as the number of children and of native-born unimmunized adults multiplied.

Smallpox caused such a scare in 1696 that the assembly, in session at Jamestown, asked for a recess—another example of the influence of disease upon political history. Earlier, in 1667, a sailor with smallpox, if the contemporary account can be accepted, landed at Accomack and was solely responsible for the outbreak of a terrible epidemic on the Eastern Shore of Virginia. A measles epidemic during the last decade of the century may actually have been smallpox as the two diseases were often confused by contemporaries.

Respiratory disorders, as has been noted, caused much distress for great numbers of early Virginians during the winter months. Influenza, pneumonia, and pleurisy must have reached epidemic proportions on numerous occasions in Virginia as elsewhere in America (influenza epidemics are recorded for New England in 1647 and in 1697-99). One note from a Virginia source for the year 1688 describes "a fast for the great mortality (the first time the winter distemper was soe very fatal... the people dyed, 1688, as in a plague... bleeding the remedy, Ld Howard had 80 ounces taken from him...)." (If "Ld Howard" gave eighty ounces, it means that he lost five pints of blood from a body that contained approximately ten—perhaps the "letting" was over an extended period.)

In a century in which numerous diseases had not been identified, many, known today, must have occurred that were diagnosed in general terms. Appendicitis, unrecognized until later, must have been common, and heart disease probably went undiagnosed. Distemper, a general term, often was used when the physician could not be more specific ("curing Eliza Mayberry and her daughter of the distemper").

Other prevalent disorders were over-eating ("hee died of a surfeit"); epilepsy ("desperately afflicted with the falling sicknesse soe that he requires continuall attendance"); and the winter cold ("our little boy & Molly have been both sicke with fever & colds, but are I thanke God now somewhat better").

The continued presence of deadly disease throughout the century shows itself in the population figures for the period. Over 100,000 persons migrated to Virginia before 1700 and numerous children were born, but only 75,000 people lived in Virginia in 1700. Many returned to Europe, many emigrated to other parts of America, and Indians accounted for some deaths, but the chief reason for the decline in population was the high mortality prevailing throughout the century.

Health conditions, however, did not deteriorate as the century passed. By 1671 Governor Berkeley could report generally improved health conditions; for example, newcomers rarely failed to survive the first few months, or seasoning period, which had formerly exacted such an awful toll. How much these improved conditions were due to better provisioned ships, to a better diet in Virginia, and to the movement of the settlers out from Jamestown is open to question, but in any consideration of the explanations for the promotion of health, prevention of illness, the restoration of health, and the rehabilitation of the sick, the seventeenth-century Virginia physician or surgeon must be considered.

PHYSICIANS AND SURGEONS IN SEVENTEENTH-CENTURY VIRGINIA

The first English medical man to set foot on Virginia soil visited the Chesapeake Bay area in 1603. Henry Kenton, a surgeon attached to a fleet exploring Virginia waters, joined the landing party that perished to a man at the hands of the Indians. Next to arrive in Virginia were the two surgeons who accompanied the first settlers in 1607 and attended their medical needs.

One of these, Thomas Wotton, was classed as a gentleman, while the other, Will Wilkinson, was listed with the laborers and craftsmen, a reminder of the varied social backgrounds of surgeons. Captain John Smith complimented Wotton in the summer of 1607 for skillful diligence in treating the sick; but Edward Maria Wingfield, when council president at Jamestown, criticized him for remaining aboard ship when the need for him ashore was so great. Because of this reputed slothfulness, Wingfield would not authorize funds for Wotton to purchase drugs and other necessaries. The colony could only have suffered from such a misunderstanding.

Further activities of Wotton and Wilkinson have faded into the mist of time past, but Captain John Smith recorded for posterity the names and deeds of other surgeons and physicians who came to Virginia before 1609. Dr. Walter Russell, the first physician—as distinguished from surgeon—to arrive, came with a contingent of new settlers and supplies in January, 1608. Post Ginnat, a surgeon, and two apothecaries, Thomas Field and John Harford, accompanied the physician. Also in Smith's record is the name, Anthony Bagnall, who has been identified as a surgeon and who came with the first supply.

Unfortunately, neither contemporaries of Russell, Ginnat, Field, and Harford—nor the men themselves—found reason to record the medical assistance they rendered during a time of great need. Russell is remembered only for the assistance he gave Smith when the Captain was severely wounded by a stingray, Post Ginnat and the apothecaries leave their names only, and Bagnall is remembered for his part in the adventures encountered on one of Captain Smith's exploratory journeys.

Russell's services to Smith deserved note because the Captain was expected to die from the stingray wound. It is an interesting comment on the medicine of the time that Smith's companions prepared his grave within four hours after the accident. "Yet by the helpe of a precious oile, Doctour Russel applyed, ere night his tormenting paine was so wel asswaged that he eate the fish to his supper."

The same stingray also assured the surgeon Bagnall a place in history. Mention of Bagnall by Captain Smith followed the surgeon's exploits on another expedition when he went along to treat the Captain's same stingray wound. The party, attacked by savages, shot one Indian in the knee and "our chirurgian ... so dressed this salvage that within an hour he looked somewhat chearfully and did eate and speake."

How unfortunate that other exploits of these physicians and surgeons, not involving Captain Smith—or the stingray—did not cause him to make a record. Dr. Lawrence Bohun, however, who accompanied Lord De la Warr to the colony in 1610, evoked comments of a more general nature in the accounts of contemporaries.

Dr. Bohun ministered to the settlers who had been ready to abandon Jamestown in 1610. A letter from the governor and council to the London Company, July 7, 1610, describes his problems and his efforts to meet them. Insomuch as the letter gives one of the fullest accounts of early Jamestown medical practices and because Bohun is one of the most renowned of seventeenth-century Virginia physicians, it deserves a lengthy quotation:

Mr. Dr. Boone [Bohun] whose care and industrie for the preservation of our men's lives (assaulted with strange fluxes and agues), we have just cause to commend unto your noble favours; nor let it, I beseech yee, be passed over as a motion slight and of no moment to furnish us with these things ... since we have true experience how many men's lives these physicke helpes have preserved since our coming, God so blessing the practise and diligence of our doctor, whose store has nowe growne thereby to so low an ebb, as we have not above 3 weekes phisicall provisions; if our men continew still thus visited with the sicknesses of the countrie, of the which every season hath his particular infirmities reigning in it, as we have it related unto us by the old inhabitants; and since our owne arrivall, have cause to feare it to be true, who have had 150 at a time much afflicted, and I am perswaded had lost the greatest part of them, if we had not brought these helpes with us.

Dr. Bohun sought medical supplies from abroad, but he also experimented with indigenous natural matter such as plants and earths in an effort to replenish his dwindling supplies and to discover natural products of value in the New World. Judging by a contemporary account, Bohun, professionally trained in the Netherlands, used drugs therapeutically according to the conventional theories of the humoral school. Despite the disfavor in which frequent purgings are held today, it must be allowed that those being treated then sounded a plaintive call for more of Bohun's "physicke."

The colony lost his services when he left to accompany Lord De la Warr to the West Indies. His connection with the London Company and its colony did not lapse, however, for Bohun received an appointment as physician-general for the colony in December, 1620. At sea, on the way to fill his post, the physician-general found his ship engaged with two Spanish men-of-war.

In the course of battle, an enemy shot mortally wounded the man who had survived great hazards at Jamestown.

After the departure of Bohun with Lord De la Warr, no physician or surgeon of equal stature or reputation took up residence in Virginia until Dr. John Pott arrived almost ten years later. It is likely that there was a shortage not only of outstanding medical men during these years, but also of medical assistance in general. Sir Thomas Dale, acting as deputy governor in the absence of De la Warr, wrote in the spring of 1611 that "our wante likewise of able chirurgions is not a little." Other requests for physicians and for apothecaries were dispatched to the London Company during this period.

However, despite the seeming shortage of medical assistance, the colonists survived such disorders as the summer seasoning much more frequently than in the first years at Jamestown. An account of Virginia written between 1616 and 1618 noted of the settlers that:

They have fallen sick, yet have recovered agayne, by very small meanes, without helpe of fresh diet, or comfort of wholsome phisique, there being at the first but few phisique helpes, or skilful surgeons, who knew how to apply the right medecine in a new country, or to search the quality and constitution of the patient, and his distemper, or that knew how to councell, when to lett blood, or not, or in necessity to use a launce in that office at all.

Bohun died in March, 1621, and the Company named his successor as physician to the colony in July. The conditions under which Dr. John Pott accepted the post reveal the qualifications and needs of the seventeenth-century medical man on his way to the New World, and the inducements offered by the Company. He was a Cambridge Master of Arts and claimed much experience in the practice of surgery and "phisique." In addition, he made much of his expertness in the distilling of water. The company allowed Pott a chest of medical supplies, a small library of medical books, and provisions for the free passage of one or more surgeons if they could be secured.

Additional economic inducements helped persuade Pott—and other physicians—to make the arduous journey to America. In the eyes of the Company, physicians could render especially valuable services to the colony, and ranked with other persons of extraordinary talent such as ministers, governors, state officers, officers of justice, and knights. These individuals received special compensations in the form of land and profits, in accord with the estimated value of services to be rendered. In 1620, Dr. Bohun had had a promise—for taking the position of physician-general for the colony—

of an allotment of 500 acres of land and ten servants; Pott accepted the job under about the same conditions as had Bohun.

These inducements offered physicians to persuade them to go to Virginia indicate the great need for, and the high value attached to, their assistance in the seventeenth century. With the population in the colony growing so great Dr. Pott's services were in considerable demand; several years after his arrival a certain William Bennett built the doctor a boat as he by then had a relatively large area to cover and most of the outlying plantations stood on the rivers and creeks.

In the colony, Pott won recognition for his professional proficiency. Even a political enemy, Governor Harvey, described him as skilled in the diagnosis and therapy of epidemic diseases. Because he alone in the colony was considered capable of treating epidemic diseases, a court sentence against him for cattle theft stood suspended early in the 1630's and clemency was sought on his behalf.

Pott had become involved in other legal difficulties before 1630. In 1625, a case having medical and humorous implications brought him into court. A Mrs. Blany maintained that Doctor Pott had denied her a piece of hog flesh, and that his refusal had caused her to miscarry. The court accepted Mrs. Blany's contention that she believed the denial of the hog flesh caused her distress, but did not hold Pott guilty of willful neglect.

Since the biographical material on Pott's non-professional life reveals so many intellectual and political interests, it would be surprising if he had not occasionally neglected his medical practice. He gave considerable time to the colony's administration and he served in 1629 as the elected temporary governor of the colony after having previously been on the governor's council. His activities in politics and affairs brought him political enemies and explain, in part, the cattle theft charge and the court's finding of "guilty" (although this was later found "rigorous if not erroneous"). He died in 1642, having been intimately involved in the life of the colony for twenty years.

Pott was the last of the outstanding figures who practiced medicine under the direction of the Company, but Dr. Wyndham B. Blanton has found mention of over 200 persons who served as physicians or surgeons during some portion of the century. With only one exception, however, none of these achieved as prominent a place in history as Bohun, Russell, or Pott. Not only is the number of outstanding individuals in the field of medicine less, but the general quality of medical practice, in the opinion of Dr. Blanton, was not as high again during the last three-quarters of the seventeenth century as it had been during the administration of the Company (1607-1624) when Virginia medicine included a representative cross-section of English medicine.

Any survey—no matter how brief—of the medical profession during the century, however, should include mention of a man who, although not a full-time professional physician, proves to be the exception to Dr. Blanton's generalization about the prominence of individual medical men and the quality of medical practice during the late 1600's. This man, the Reverend John Clayton, is a noteworthy example of the intellectual level an individual could attain and maintain while living in an area that was still remote from European civilization.

Clayton, who is known to have been at Jamestown between 1684 and 1686 as a clergyman, also practiced medicine in addition to pursuing his scientific interests. As a prolific writer he has left some of the fullest and most interesting accounts of contemporary treatment and diagnosis. His knowledge and methods cannot be taken as typical, however, because his intellectual level was considerably above the average in the colony.

This minister-scientist-physician wrote an account of his treatment of a case of hydrophobia resulting from the bite of a rabid dog. With its accomplished style, Clayton's account of his treatment of hydrophobia is worthy of attention as an example of contemporary theory and practice of the more learned kind. He wrote:

It was a relapse of its former distemper, that is, of the bite of the mad-dog. I told them, if any thing in the world would save his life, I judged it might be the former vomit of volatile salts; they could not tell what to do, nevertheless such is the malignancy of the world, that as soon as it was given, they ran away and left me, saying, he was now certainly a dead man, to have a vomit given in that condition. Nevertheless it pleased God that he shortly after cried, *this fellow in the black has done me good*, and after the first vomit, came so to himself, as to know us all.

Subsequently, Clayton "vomited him" every other day and made him take volatile salt of amber between vomitings. The patient also drank "posset-drink" with "sage and rue," and washed his hands and sores in a strong salt brine. Cured by the "fellow in the black," the patient had no relapse.

Clayton reveals more of his medical theory in another passage from his writings. He observed:

In September the weather usually breaks suddenly, and there falls generally very considerable rains. When the weather breaks many fall sick, this being the time of an endemical sickness, for seasonings, cachexes, fluxes, scorbutical dropsies, gripes, or the like which I have attributed to this reason. That by the extraordinary heat, the ferment of the blood being raised too high, and the tone of the stomach relaxed, when the weather breaks the blood palls, and like overfermented liquors is depauperated, or turns eager and sharp, and there's a crude digestion, whence the name distempers may be supposed to ensue.

In this passage Clayton's medical theory resembles closely the orthodox medical beliefs of the century. The great English practitioner Sydenham, for example, emphasized the relationship between the weather and disease. Also the analogy between the behavior of blood and wine was then conventional, and the supposed connection between the "sour" blood and indigestion with the resulting acid humors is in accord with Galenism. The remedy—and a most logical one—was medicine to combat the acidity and to restore the tone or balance to the stomach. Acid stomach has a long history.

The reasonableness of Clayton's pathology is impressive, but reason did lead to some bizarre—in the light of present-day medical knowledge— conclusions. Aware of the value to the scientist of close observation and of the necessity to reason about these observations, Clayton was in the finest seventeenth-century scientific tradition. Observing a lady—for example— suffering from lead poisoning, he noted that her distress, judging by her behavior, varied directly with the nearness and bigness of the passing clouds; the nearer the clouds, the more anguished her groans. Reason dictated to Clayton that such a phenomenon stemmed from a cause-effect relationship.

Although the twentieth-century physician would deny the cloud-suffering association, he would not deny Clayton's propensity for observation and his attempts to discern relationships. The approach of the better seventeenth-century Virginia physician can be labeled scientific even if his facts were few.

DRUGS AND OTHER REMEDIES

No seventeenth-century physician could function without a variety of drugs (medicines) to dispense. Dr. Pott made special arrangements—for example—to have a chest of drugs transported with him from England to America, and the effectiveness of Dr. Bohun's "physicke" drew the praise of the colonists. Drugs were essential to the physician and a valuable commodity for export, as well. The subject of drugs must then include a discussion of their use as medicines and their importance as items of trade.

A study of the drugs in use and the occasions of their utilization makes manifest the great part that freeing the body from corrupting matter played in the treatment of disease. The theorists and clinical physicians of the century placed such faith in the humoral doctrine that, on the basis of this predilection, much of the opposition to cinchona, or quinine, in a period greatly troubled by malaria, can be explained. Cinchona, discovered in Spanish America and known in seventeenth-century Europe, had demonstrable effects in the treatment of malaria but, because it was an additive rather than a purgative, physicians rejected it on theoretical grounds. Its eventual acceptance later revolutionized drug therapeutics, but this revolution did not affect seventeenth-century Virginia.

The emphasis that the contemporary medical men placed upon the purging of the body—the vomiting, sweating, purgings of the bowels, the draining, and the bleeding—cannot be considered irrational or quaint. In the light of observation and common sense, to purge seemed not only reasonable and natural but in accord with orthodox doctrine as well. Observation revealed that illness was frequently accompanied by an excess of fluid or matter in the body, as in the case of colds, respiratory disorders, swollen joints, diarrheas, or the skin eruptions that accompanied such epidemic diseases as the plague or smallpox. Common sense dictated a freeing of the body of the corrupt or corrupting matter; drugs were a means to this end.

The use of drugs for vomiting, sweating, and other forms of purging seems excessive in the light of present-day medical knowledge, and at least one seventeenth-century Virginia student of medicine also found such use of drugs by his contemporaries open to criticism. In the opinion of the Reverend John Clayton, Virginia doctors were so prone to associate all drugs with vomiting or other forms of purging that they even thought of aromatic spirits as an inferior "vomitive." He concluded that these physicians would purge violently even for an aching finger: "they immediately [upon examining the patients] give three or four spoonfuls [of *crocus metallorum*] ... then perhaps purge them with fifteen or twenty grains of the rosin of jalap, afterwards sweat them with Venice treacle, powder of snakeroot, or Gascoin's Powder; and when these fail *conclamatum est.*"

The list of drugs used was extensive and each drug had a considerable literature written about it explaining the various sicknesses and disorders for which it was a curative. Libraries of the Virginia physicians and of the well-to-do laymen usually included a volume or two on the use of drugs. Among the most popular plants, roots, and other natural products were snakeroot, dittany, senna, alum, sweet gums, and tobacco.

Dittany drove worms out of the body and would also produce sweat (sweating being another popular method of purging the body of disease-producing matter). The juices of the fever or ague-root in beer or water "purgeth downward with some violence ... in powder ... it only moveth sweat." (Following Galen's system of classifying by taste, this root was bitter, therefore thought dry. The physician would administer such a drying agent when attempting to reduce excess moistness in the body—and thus restore normal body balance, in accord with contemporary humoral theory.) Snakeroot, another of the popular therapeutics, increased the output of urine and of perspiration; black snakeroot, remedying rheumatism, gout, and amenorrhea, found such wide usage during the last half of the seventeenth century that its price per pound in Virginia on one occasion rose from ten shillings to three pounds sterling. Although King James I of England saw much danger in tobacco, others among his subjects attributed phenomenal curative properties to it. One late sixteenth-century commentator on America recommended it as a purge for superfluous phlegm; and smokers believed it functioned as an antidote for poisons, as an expellant for "sour" humors, and as a healer of wounds. Some doctors maintained that it would heal gout and the ague, act as a stimulant and appetite depressant, and counteract drunkenness.

The full significance of these drugs in the medicine of the period can be better appreciated by reference to a prescription for their use, in this instance a remedy for rickets, thought typical by historian Thomas Jefferson Wertenbaker:

Dip the child in the morning, head foremost in cold water, don't dress it immediately, but let it be made warm in the cradle & sweat at least half an hour moderately. Do this 3 mornings ... & if one or both feet are cold while other parts sweat let a little blood be taken out of the feet the 2nd morning.... Before the dips of the child give it some snakeroot and saffern steep'd in rum & water, give this immediately before diping and after you have dipt the child 3 mornings. Give it several times a day the following syrup made of comfry, hartshorn, red roses, hog-brake roots, knot-grass, petty-moral roots; sweeten the syrup with melosses.

But drug therapy was not always as simple as that recommended for rickets, although the evidence is that in Virginia the high cost of importing the rarer substances inclined local physicians toward the less elaborate compounds. Venice treacle, recommended by the Reverend Clayton's imaginary purge enthusiast consisted of vipers, white wine, opium, licorice, red roses, St. John's wort, and at least a half-dozen other ingredients.

Because their use was so extensive in Europe and because many brought a good price, any discussion of drugs in seventeenth-century Virginia should take note of the efforts in the colony to find locally the raw materials for the drugs both for use in Virginia and for export. The London Company actively supported a program to develop the drug resources of the New World, and the hope of finding them had originally been one of the incentives for the colonization of Virginia. Even as early as the sixteenth century, authors and promoters in England of the American venture had held up the promise of a profitable trade in drugs—sassafras, for example—as a stimulus for exploration and colonization. Sassafras had market value as it was widely used in cases of dysentery, skin diseases, and as a stimulant and astringent; French warships searching for loot off the shores of the New World had often made it the cargo when richer prizes were not to be had.

Like gold, sassafras diverted labor during the crucial early period at Jamestown from the tasks of building and provisioning. Sailors and settlers, both, took time off to load the ships with the drug which would bring a good price in England.

The belief that the exporting of drugs would prove profitable for the colony in Virginia and for the Company may explain why two apothecaries accompanied the second group of immigrants who arrived in 1608. Someone had to search out and identify possible drugs, and a layman could not be expected to perform a task requiring such specialized knowledge. The apothecaries could further serve the new settlement by helping to supply its medicinal needs.

Before the drug trade in Virginia could be developed, and at the same time adapted to the over-all needs of the colony, attention had to be given to the use of drugs to meet the immediate needs of the settlers. Dr. Bohun, who had brought medical supplies in 1610 and soon found them exhausted, turned resourcefully to an investigation of indigenous minerals and plants. He investigated earths, gums, plants, and fruits. A white clay proved useful in treating the fevers (the clay of the Indians used for "sicknesse and paine of the belly"?); the fruits of a tree similar to the "mirtle" helped the doctor to face the epidemics of dysentery.

The colonists also needed a wine which could be produced cheaply and locally. Many of them, accustomed to beer and wine regularly, complained of having to rely upon water as a liquid refresher. According to one of their number, more died in Virginia of the "disease of their minds than of their body ... and by not knowing they shall drink water here." One enterprising alchemist and chemist offered to sell the London Company a solution for this problem: the formula of an artificial wine to be made from Virginia vegetables.

After the colony seemed no longer in danger of perishing from its own sicknesses—or going mad from having to drink water—the Company urged the settlers to develop an active trade in medicinal plants, in order to help cure the diseases of England and the financial ills of the Company. The London Company, in a carefully organized memorandum, advised the colonists what plants had export value and how these plants should be prepared for export:

1. Small sassafras rootes to be drawen in the winter and dryed and none to be medled with in the sommer, and it is worthe 50 lb. and better per tonne.

2. Poccone to be gotten from the Indians and put up in caske is worthe per tonne 11 lb. 4. Galbrand groweth like fennell in fashion, and there is greatest stoare of it in Warriscoes Country, where they cut walnut trees leaste. You must cut it downe in Maye or June, and beinge downe it is to be cut into small peeces, and brused and pressed in your small presses, the juice thereof is to be saved and put into casks, which wilbe worthe here per tonne, 100 lb. at leasts. 5. Sarsapilla is a roote that runneth within the grounds like unto licoras, which beareth a small rounde leafe close by the grounds, which being founde the roote is to be pulled up and dryed and bounde up in bundles like faggotts, this is to be done towards the ende of sommer before the leafe fall from the stalk; and it is worthe here per tonne, 200 lb. 6. Wallnutt oyle is worth here 30 lb. per tonne, and the like is chestnutt oyle and chechinkamyne oyle.

The Company's plan for the gathering, storing, and shipping of drugs was supplemented by a project indicating foresight and an early form of experimental research for the development of new products. In 1621 it planned thorough tests of an earth sent from Virginia in order to determine its value as a cure for the flux. In addition, the Company planned to test all sweet gums, roots, woods, and berries submitted by the colonists in order to ascertain their medicinal values.

In regard to the sale and dispensing of drugs in Virginia, whether found locally or imported, frequent references to the apothecary supplies and utensils in the possession of Virginia physicians lead to the conclusion that they were usually their own druggists.

As has been noted, the sale and dispensing of drugs usually culminated in their use—in accordance with the theory of the period—as means of purging the body. Drugs, however, did not have a monopoly in this greatly emphasized aspect of medical practice because the clyster (purging of the bowels, or enema) and phlebotomy (bleeding of the vein) could be used as well. These two methods might be classified as mechanical in nature as contrasted with the essentially chemical action of the drugs.

Molière, in his seventeenth-century satires on the European medical profession, ridicules the excessive use of the clyster. The popularity of the phlebotomy then is attested to by the notoriety of this technique today. (Rare is the schoolboy who does not think that George Washington was bled to death.) There is no reason to doubt that the clyster and phlebotomy enjoyed as wide usage in colonial Virginia as in Europe, but the evidence surviving to prove this assumption is slight.

Dr. Blanton, the historian of medicine, could find only meager references to the use of clyster (or glyster) and he sums them up as follows:

Among the effects of Nathaniel Hill was '1 old syringe.' In York County records we find that Thomas Whitehead in 1660 paid Edmond Smith for '2 glysters.' George Wale's account to the estate of Thomas Baxter in 1658 included a similar charge. George Light in 1657 paid Dr. Modè fifty pounds of tobacco for 'a glister and administering.' John Clulo, Francis Haddon and William Lee each presented bills for similar services.

The survival of such meager evidence for what was probably a common practice indicates the difficulties confronting the historian of medicine. Nor has Dr. Blanton been able to find, as a result of his research, any more evidence of phlebotomy although, again, its utilization must have been widespread. Blanton sums up his evidence for bleeding as follows:

Dr. Modé's bill to George Light includes 'a phlebothany to Jno Simonds' and 'a phlebothany to yr mayd.' Dr. Henry Power twice bled Thomas Cowell of York County in 1680, and Patrick Napier twice phlebotomized 'Allen Jarves, deceased, in the cure of a cancer of his mouth.' Colonel Daniel Parke in 1665 rendered John Horsington a bill for 'lettinge blood' from his servant; and we find Dr. Jeremiah Rawlins and Francis Haddon engaging in the same practice.

The horoscope often determined the proper time for bleeding and notations have been found in an early American Bible recommending the days to, and not to, bleed. Although medicine today looks askance at astrological medicine and bloodletting, it remains difficult to explain the widespread popularity of such practices unless the patients enjoyed some beneficial results, psychological or physical.

Drug therapeutics, clysters, and bloodletting did by no means exhaust the seventeenth-century physician's treatments and remedies. The works of European painters of the century remind us of uroscopy or urine examination. One of the outstanding paintings illustrating the technique is by artist Gerard Dou who has the young doctor intently examining the urine flask while taking the pulse of a pretty young lady. Unfortunately, such revealing pictorial representations of life and medicine in colonial Virginia do not exist.

On the other hand, in Virginia, the Reverend John Clayton displayed a distinct flair for the scientific method in his analysis of urine. It is safe to assume that his techniques were of a higher order than those usually associated with uroscopy. Clayton, not satisfied to practice just the art of observation, utilized the science of comparative weights hoping to find diseases distinguished by minute variations in the specific gravity of the liquid. He thought he could find manifestations of "affections in the head" by his careful weighing and study; manifestations not uncovered by visual observations alone.

In Gerard Dou's painting, it is to be remembered, the doctor not only examined the urine but also took the pulse—another common practice. This is not surprising insomuch as Galen—the great and ancient authority—had written enough to fill sixteen books on the subject of "pulse lore." Despite the facts that physicians centuries later continue to take the pulse, they would not find the theories behind the seventeenth-century practice acceptable. Galen's deductions have since been described as fantastic, and his attempt to associate a specific type of pulse rate with every disease futile. Yet the Virginia physician, when he did take his patient's pulses, certainly did not lose his or her confidence by gravely considering the mysterious palpitation.

The physician with his many techniques and remedies did not restrict himself solely to the illnesses of the sane for—contrary to popular belief today—some effort was made to treat and cure the mentally ill. America's first insane asylum was not established until 1769, but the insane had received, even before this, medical attention. If the case did not respond to treatment and took a turn toward violence, confinement under conditions that would now be considered barbarous often resulted. Before this extreme solution of an extreme problem recommended itself, however, the mentally ill might be purged. The intent was to relieve the patient of insanity-producing yellow and black bile. The belief that this type of sickness would respond to conventional treatment, however, did not completely dominate the theories on insanity; some seventeenth-century authorities considered insanity not an illness but an incurable, disgraceful condition.

One of the fullest accounts of a case of insanity in seventeenth-century Virginia describes the plight of poor John Stock of York who kept "running about the neighborhood day and night in a sad distracted condition to the great disturbance of the people." The court authorities ordered that Stock be confined but provided such "helps as may be convenient to looke after him." The court, in a sanguine mood, anticipated the day when Stock would be in a better condition to govern himself.

HOUSING OF THE SICK

If the doctor, surgeon, or nursing persons could come to the patient's home, little advantage could have been obtained in the seventeenth century by moving the patient. The need did arise, however, to care for persons outside the home. For example, an individual without family or close friends might find it more convenient to move in with those who would care for him on a professional basis, or newly arrived immigrants and transients might need housing.

Quite in harmony with the needs of the period were the men and women willing to take in a sick person in order to supplement their incomes. Illness forced one colonial Virginian to offer in 1686 to grant his plantation and his home to the person who would provide a wholesome diet, washing, and lodging for him and his two daughters. The beneficiary was also to carry the sick man to a doctor and to pay all of his debts. It is probable that the man provided these services only on this particular occasion, but by such special arrangements the century housed its sick. The number of ill persons provided for by relatives under similar arrangements or even without any compensation, must have been even greater in a period without hospitals and nursing homes.

On occasions, in the seventeenth century, the physician took the patient into his own home, but not always without some reluctance. Dr. Wyndham B. Blanton, in his search of the Virginia records for this century, found an interesting account of Dr. George Lee of Surry County, Virginia, who in 1676 had an unfortunate experience in letting accommodations to a pregnant woman. Living in a house she considered open and unavoidably cold, and having only one old sow for food, the sick and feverish woman pleaded with the doctor to take her to his home for the lying-in period. The doctor argued that the house could be made warmer, suggested that neighbors bring in food, and protested that he had only one room fit for such occupancy and that he and his wife used it. Dr. Lee said he would not give up the room for anyone in Virginia.

Offering the opinion that the room was large enough for her, Dr. Lee, and his wife, the expectant mother had her servant take her by boat to Lee's where she remained, taking great quantities of medicine, until she delivered. The doctor then had to bring suit to collect his fees.

Another example of a medical man's housing the sick, is that of a surgeon promised 2,000 pounds of tobacco and "cask" if he cured the blindness of a person he had housed—but only modest compensation if he failed. The same surgeon received 1,000 pounds of tobacco in 1681 by order of the vestry of Christ Church parish for keeping "one Mary Teston, poore impotent person."

Much earlier, Virginia had what some authorities consider to be the first hospital built in America. While the colony was still under the administration of the London Company (1612), a structure was erected near the present site of Dutch Gap on the James river to house the sick. The hospital, which had provisions for medical and surgical patients, stood opposite Henrico, a thriving outpost of the settlement of Jamestown.

Evidence that the building was primarily designed for the sick and was not simply a public guest house is to be found in the statements of contemporaries. One described it as a "retreat or guest house for sicke people, a high seat and wholesome air," while another wrote that "here they were building also an hospitall with fourscore lodgings (and beds alreadie sent to furnish them) for the sicke and lame, with keepers to attend them for their comfort and recoverie." The use of the word "hospital," which had then a general sense, does not indicate any similarity to a present-day hospital as does the other information. Nothing more appears about this establishment for the sick and wounded, and it may well have been destroyed during the Indian uprising of 1622.

Plans for similar institutions in each of the major political and geographical subdivisions of the colony came from the London Company. Unlike the Henrico structure, these buildings bore the name "guest house" and were to harbor the sick and to receive strangers. Specifications called for twenty-five beds for fifty persons (which was in accord with custom in public institutions); board partitions between the beds; five conveniently placed chimneys; and windows enough to provide ample fresh air.

The Company repeatedly recommended and urged the construction of these guest houses not only as a retreat for the sick but also as a measure to prevent illness among the newcomers. In addition, the guest houses, if they had been built, would have saved the old settlers from being exposed to the diseases of the new arrivals who were taken into private homes. The colonists always had some excuse for delaying construction, and the Company in 1621 entreated to the effect that it could not "but apprehend with great grief the sufferings of these multitudes at their first landing for want of guest houses where in they might have a while sheltered themselves from the injuries of the air in the cold season."

That the London Company should have had the Henrico hospital built during its administration and made plans for the guest houses can be explained by the situation existing during the earlier days of the colony. The Company, engaged in a commercial venture and realizing by its own statement that "in the health of the people consisteth the very life, strength, increase and prosperity of the whole general colony," had sufficient reason to shelter and care for the colonists. Also, during the early days the number of incoming colonists was high relative to the number settled and with lodging to give or to let. The Company, in addition, knew that new arrivals fell victim most easily to seasoning and other maladies, and needed protection from the elements. Finally, the Company had to fill the void created by the absence of religious orders which, during prior European colonization and occupation of distant lands, had provided shelter and care. These hospitals are no longer mentioned after the dissolution of the London Company, nor were any other comparable measures taken during the century to institutionalize care for the sick.

Much has been made of the lower status held by the surgeon as compared with that of the physician—during the seventeenth century. On the continent and in England, at this period, membership in separate guilds in part distinguished doctor and surgeon; in England, after 1540 and until 1745, surgeons held common membership with barbers in one corporate organization. In America, historians agree, the differences based on specialization of practice between surgeons and physicians soon tended to disappear, a superior education often being the only attribute or function of a physician not shared by the surgeon. Barbers held a unique position, but in performing phlebotomies, a minor operation, they retained associations with health and disease. Both barber and surgeon shared a certain expertness with tools, as they do today.

Evidence abounds in the earlier records that the scarcity of medical men may have compelled surgeons in Virginia to practice internal medicine: surgeons prescribed medicine with the same frequency as doctors. The surgeons, however, did not abandon the treatment of wounds, fractures, and dislocations; notes on amputations during the century also exist.

Nor is it reasonable to assume that the isolated physician of the Virginia countryside would always insist upon referring a patient to a surgeon. Dr. Francis Haddon, who had a large practice in York County, Virginia, and who is not identified as a surgeon, left recorded the course of treatment for an amputation—cordials, a purge, ointments, and bloodletting—and a dismembering saw, as well.

Other recorded surgical treatments include care of dislocated shoulders; wounds in various parts of the body; sores of the feet and legs; cancerous ulcers in the instep; ulcers of the throat, and dueling wounds. One of the most unusual surgical measures of the period was the application of weapon salve for battle wounds; the salve was applied to weapon, not wound.

Surgery has long been associated with the military, and much of the outstanding surgical work done in Europe during the fifteenth and sixteenth centuries was performed by military surgeons. Ambroise Paré (c. 1510-1590), remembered especially for the use of the ligature in amputations and the abandonment of the burning-oil treatment of wounds, held a position as a surgeon for the French army. Other surgeons of the period contributed to the improvement of medical practice by enlightened measures of quarantine to prevent contagious diseases from decimating armies.

Insomuch as the first settlers at Jamestown greatly feared attack from Indians and Spaniards and because the initial landings had the character of a military expedition, it is not surprising that the first two medical men to arrive, Will

Wilkinson and Thomas Wotton, were surgeons. Captain John Smith on three occasions, it is to be remembered, emphasized the importance of the surgeon to pioneer settlers and explorers in the New World. When injured by the stingray in 1608, Smith's first thought was of his need for a surgeon and "chirurgery"; so the success of physician Russell's soothing oils came as a pleasant surprise. On a subsequent expedition he included the surgeon, Anthony Bagnall, rather than Dr. Russell, to treat the stingray wound; and in 1609 when he received the powder burn, he left Virginia "seeing there was neither chirurgeon nor chirurgery in the fort to cure his hurt."

Throughout the century surgeons rendered services to colonists engaged in fighting with, or defending themselves against, the Indians. When the Indian massacre of 1622 occurred, costing the lives of more than 350 colonists in the settlements, it is possible that the two surgeons who sailed to Virginia with Dr. Pott in 1621 gave assistance to the wounded. In 1644, when a retaliatory attack on the Indians was made by the settlers because of a recent massacre, the General Assembly provided for a surgeon-general to accompany the militia, at public expense.

Again, later in the century, the General Assembly gave evidence of recognizing the importance of surgical care for soldiers when it voted for supplying a surgeon with "a convenient supply of medicines & salves, etc. to the value of five pounds sterling for every hundred men" to each of eight forts planned to protect the settlements against Indian attacks. Throughout the last half of the century references were made to surgeons ministering to companies of soldiers or to various garrisons and forts. Judging by the consistent employment of surgeons for military duties, it would appear that the profession of surgeon during the century was much more intimately associated with the military than was that of physician. The relationship between the surgeon and the military is similar to the early one between civil engineer and the army in Europe.

HYGIENE

The restoration of the patient to health is not the only important aspect of medical practice; the prevention of illness is also vital to the health of a community. Much more attention is given to preventive medicine in the twentieth century than in the seventeenth, but the value of cleanliness, fresh air, and quarantine was known. Hygienic measures taken, or recommendations made, by public authorities make clear the fact that the cause of disease was not commonly thought to be supernatural by the educated and responsible. Contemporary accounts make known the widespread disapproval of foul ships, crowded quarters, marshy land, stagnant air, bad food and drink, excessive eating, and exposure to a hot sun.

Lord De la Warr laid down regulations for Jamestown designed to eliminate the dangers of dirty wash water ("no ... water or suds of fowle cloathes or kettle, pot, or pan ... within twenty foote of the olde well"); and of contamination from sewage ("nor shall any one aforesaid, within lesse than a quarter of one mile from the pallisadoes, dare to doe the necessities of nature"). The order argued that if the inhabitants did not separate themselves at least a quarter of one mile from the palisaded living area that "the whole fort may be choaked, and poisoned with ill aires and so corrupt." The colonists by the same order had to keep their own houses and the street before both sweet and clean.

Any doubt that an awareness existed of the dangers of infection by contact, at least from diseases with observable bodily symptoms, should be dispelled by the quarantine measures taken by the colonel and commander of Northampton County in 1667 during an epidemic of smallpox. He ordered that no member of a family inflicted with the disease should leave his house until thirty days after the outbreak lest the disease be spread by infection "like the plague of leprosy." Enlightened authorities in Europe took similar precautions.

CHAPTER FOUR

Education, Women, Churchmen, and The Law

THE PLACE OF WOMEN IN MEDICINE

Women played a part in treating and caring for the ill and distressed in a number of ways during the century. A few women dispensed medicine and enjoyed reputations as doctors, but it was in the field of obstetrics and as midwives that they made their most important contributions. Although women did what might be described generally as nursing, their contribution in this area was relatively insignificant when compared with the importance of the female nurse today. Any discussion of the place of women in seventeenth-century medicine should note the relationship between women, witchcraft, and medicine.

Although the references leave no doubt of the existence of female doctors and dispensers of medicines, the mention of them is infrequent. Mrs. Mary Seal, the widow of a Dr. Power, for example, administered medicine to Richard Dunbar in 1700. The wife of Edward Good was sought out in 1678 to cure a head sore and another "doctress" impressed the Reverend John Clayton, who had some insights into medical science himself, with her ability to cure the bite of a rattlesnake by using the drug dittany. In the same year that Good's wife was sought to treat the head sore, a Mrs. Grendon dispensed medicine to an individual who had injured his eyes in a fight. The exact status of these women, however, is unknown; it is highly unlikely that the female practicing medicine enjoyed the professional standing of a Dr. Pott or a Dr. Bohun—an old female slave also appears in the record as a doctor.

With medical knowledge limited and antisepsis unknown, the expectant mother of the seventeenth century fared better with a midwife than she would have with a physician. The midwife, whose training consisted of experience and apprenticeship at best, allowed the birth to be as free from human interference as possible and did not do a pre-delivery infection-producing examination.

Both the fees and the prestige of the midwife, judging by contemporary records from other colonies, were high. Unfortunately, the early Virginia sources throw little light on the activities of the midwife in this colony. Among the scattered references from Virginia records are found charges of 100 pounds of tobacco for the service of a midwife; the presence of two midwives assisted by two nurses and other women at a single birth; the payment of twelve hens for obstetrical services; and the delivery of a bastard child by a midwife.

Nursing duties were probably taken on by both men and women in addition to their regular occupations. The duties consisted not only of tending the sick—and there is no reason to believe this was done under the supervision of a physician—but also of burying the dead and arranging the funerals. While the patient lived, the nurse prepared food, washed linen, and did other chores to make the patient comfortable. When death came, the nurse was "the good woman who shall dress me and put me in my coffin," and who provided "entertainment of those that came to bury him with 3 vollys of shott & diging his grave with the trouble of his funeral included."

The medical ramifications of witchcraft have been suggested. One of the most interesting Virginia court cases of the century had as its principal subject a woman accused of the power to cause sickness. In an age when weapon salve was wiped on the weapon and not the wound, and when astrology was intimately associated with the practice of medicine, it is not surprising to find, also, the witch and her power to cause disease. Goodwife Wright stood accused of such powers in the colony's general court on September 11, 1626.

Goodwife Wright had caused, according to her accusers, the illness of a husband, wife, and child out of a spirit of revenge; and she was able to prophesy deaths as well. The details of the case brought against this woman accused of witchcraft reveal the more bizarre medical practices of the time. Goodwife Wright expected to serve as the midwife but the expectant mother refused to employ her upon learning that Wright was left-handed. Soon after affronting Wright in such a manner, the mother complained that her breast "grew dangerouslie sore" and her husband and child both fell sick within a few weeks. With circumstantial evidence of this kind, suspicion had little difficulty in linking the midwife with the sicknesses.

Testimony revealed that on another occasion she had used her powers to counter the actions of another suspected witch. Having been informed that the other witch was causing the sickness, Wright had the ill person throw a red-hot horseshoe into her own urine. The result, according to witnesses was that the offending witch was "sick at harte" as long as the horseshoe was hot, and the sick person well when it had cooled.

CHURCHMEN AND MEDICINE

Medicine was associated in many minds not only with the powers of evil but also with the forces for good. The clergyman in colonial America often practiced medicine, and the layman in some localities of Virginia could turn to the local parson for medical assistance.

Throughout the early Christian era and the medieval period, medicine and religion had had a close relationship. The New Testament had numerous references to the healing of the sick by spiritual means, and a casual relationship between sin and physical affliction had been assumed by many persons for centuries before the seventeenth. The hand of God was still seen by many in physical phenomena, whether disease or the flight of a comet. Not only was there a supernatural relationship seen between the God of the church and disease, but also a natural one between medicine and the church clergy, for they had staffed the medical schools for centuries. It is not surprising, then, that the parson-physician was no stranger to the Virginia colony.

As early as 1619, Robert Pawlett, known to be a preacher, surgeon, and physician, came to Virginia. He was followed by other parson-physicians in Virginia and in other colonies. As late as the end of the eighteenth century, the wife of George Washington called on the Reverend Greene, M.D., for medical advice.

Among the most interesting in this long tradition of ministers who practiced medicine is the Reverend John Clayton whose activities have been noted. Other persons residing in Virginia and combining the role of clergyman with a considerable interest in medicine were Nathaniel Eaton, who had a degree in medicine, and John Banister who was an active naturalist. As a naturalist, he made an important study of the plants of Virginia (*Catalogue of Virginia Plants*) which added to the literature available for the dispenser of medicinal drugs. One of the founders of Presbyterianism in America, the Reverend Francis Makemie, who came to America in 1681 and died in Accomack County, Virginia, was described as a preacher, a doctor of medicine, a merchant, an attorney—and a disturber of government by the governor of New York.

LAW AND MEDICINE

Although the Crown did not follow the lead of the Company in providing care for the sick and unsheltered, the authorities after 1624 did have the state take an interest in medicine to the extent of passing laws dealing with medical problems and situations. These laws were primarily concerned with the collection and charging of fees, but also provided for the censure of the physician or surgeon neglecting his patient.

On four occasions during the century the Assembly attempted to regulate the excessive and immoderate rates of physicians and surgeons. The chief example used to convey the injustice of fees for visits and drugs was that many colonists preferred to allow their servants to hazard a recovery than to call a medical man. Although an inhumane attitude, the colonists reasoned that the physician or surgeon would charge more than the purchase price of the servant.

The act of 1657-58 reveals this attitude and throws some light on the medical practice of the century. (Similar acts had been passed in 1639 and in 1645 and would be passed in 1661-62.) By the will of the Assembly, the layman had the right to bring the physician or surgeon into court if the charge for "paines, druggs or medicines" was thought to be unreasonable. The surgeon or physician had in court to declare under oath the true value of drugs and medicines administered, and then the court decided the just compensation.

The law went on to declare that:

Where it shall be sufficiently proved in any of the said courts that a phisitian or chirurgeon hath neglected his patient, or that he hath refused (being thereunto required) his helpe and assistance to any person or persons in sicknes or extremitie, that the said phisitian or chirurgeon shall be censured by the court for such his neglect or refusall.

The legislators also gave the physician or surgeon protection by providing that their accounts could be pleaded against and recovered from the estate of a deceased patient—suggesting that patients were not prompt enough in paying their bills (or perhaps did not survive treatment long enough to do so). Court records show that the medical men often took advantage of this provision for collection.

A measure enacted in 1692 indicated a more sympathetic attitude on the part of the legislators toward the physicians and surgeons. While in the earlier acts preventing exorbitant fees the court had been ordered to decide upon just compensation, the later act allowed the physician or surgeon to charge whatever he declared under oath in court to be just for medicines. Nor did the act of 1692 make reference to "rigorous though unskilful" or "griping and avaricious" physicians and surgeons as had the earlier laws.

References by the colonial Assembly to exorbitant fees were not without a basis in fact. The conventional charge for the physician's visit, according to Dr. Wyndham Blanton, was thirty-five to fifty pounds of tobacco and on occasions the physician, or surgeon, must have exceeded this fee. An approximate estimate of the value of these visits in present-day terms would be between twenty and twenty-five dollars. The cost of medical care was even greater when an unusually large amount of drugs was dispensed. It is not surprising that many masters did not provide the services of a physician or surgeon for their servants; nor that medical attention was given by persons without professional status. Although these charges seem high, it must be taken into account that because of the great distances between communities and even between homes, the physician or surgeon could make only a small number of visits each week.

County records give many examples of the fees of physicians and surgeons. Of 145 medical bills entered in the York County records between 1637 and 1700, the average bill was for 752 pounds of tobacco, or a little less than one laborer could produce in a year. Other fees were: 400 pounds of tobacco for six visits; 300 pounds of tobacco for three visits and five days attendance; 1,000 pounds of tobacco for twenty days of attendance "going ounce a weeke ... being fourteen miles"; and 600 pounds for twelve daily visits. At the time these charges were made, tobacco brought between two and three cents per pound, or the equivalent of approximately fifty cents today.

The surgeon administering the clyster or phlebotomy, those commonly resorted to "remedies," could be expected to charge thirty pounds of tobacco for the first and twenty pounds for the second. The surgeon, and the physician, often charged from twenty to fifty pounds of tobacco for a drug prescription.

In 1658, Dr. John Clulo presented a bill to John Gosling in York County which he itemized as follows (in pounds of tobacco):

For 2 glisters [clysters]	040
For a glister	030
For a potion cord.[ial]	036
For an astringent potion	035
For my visitts paines & attendance	...
For a glistere	030
For an astringent potion	035
For a cord. astringent bole	036
For a bole as before	036
For a purging potion	050
For a [cordial julep]	120
For a potion as before	036

Not only does Dr. Clulo's bill give examples of fees charged, but it supports the contention that the substance of medical treatment during the century was bloodletting, purging, and prescribing drugs.

Although the physicians of colonial Virginia did charge well for their services, it should be noted that they were in demand. Their patients, this would indicate, considered their services of great value, any subsequent protests notwithstanding.

THE EDUCATION OF PHYSICIANS AND SURGEONS

Since the physicians and surgeons did make substantial charges and since the educated layman could buy his own books on medicine and practice what he read or since the uneducated could turn to a neighbor with medical knowledge or to a quack, the question arises as to why the services of professional surgeons and physicians were in such demand. Part of the answer lies in the professional's experience, but even in a colony without a medical school it also lies in the education and training received by the professional.

There were several ways in which a seventeenth-century Virginia physician could acquire his education or training. He could have received a medical degree in England or on the continent and then gone to America. On the other hand, he might have learned without formal education—perhaps by attending lectures and by experience—and then established himself in Virginia where he was accorded professional status. A man born in Virginia could return to the Old World for training or formal education and then practice in Virginia. Also, a common manner of becoming a physician or surgeon in Virginia, which was without medical schools, was by apprenticeship. Finally, the importance of books—imported from Europe— as a means to medical education should not be minimized.

To be officially licensed for practice, the requirements in England were high—those in London especially so. The following excerpt from the statutes of the College of Physicians of London demonstrates how demanding the educational standards for seventeenth-century English physicians could be:

First, let them be examined in the physiologick part, and the very rudiments of medicine, and in this examination let questions be propounded out of the books concerning elements, temperaments, the use of parts, anatomy, natural powers and faculties, and other parts of natural medicine.

Secondly let him be examined in the pathologick part, or concerning the causes, differences, symptoms and signs of diseases, which physicians make use of to know the essence of diseases; and in this examination let questions be proposed out of books concerning the art of physick, of the places affected, of the differences of diseases and symptoms, of feavers, of the pubes, of the books of prognosticks of Hippocrates, &c.

Thirdly let him be examined concerning the use and exercise of medicine, or the reason of healing; and let that be done out of the books concerning preservation of health, of the method of healing, of the reason of diet in acute diseases, of simple medicines, of crises, of the aphorisms of Hyppocrates, and other things of that kind, which relate to the use of healing; for example sake, what caution to be observed in purging? in what persons? with what medicine? and in what vein, those things ought to be done? Likewise, what is the use of narcoticks and sleeping medicines? and what caution is to be observed in them? what is the position and site of the internal places? and by what passages medicines come to there? what is the use of clysters, what kind of vomits, the danger, kind and measure?

Under the London Company, the physicians and surgeons in Virginia had the same education, training, and met the same standards as their counterparts in England. This was, in part, because the Company had good reason to supply adequate medical service, and because the men sent were but Englishmen transplanted to America. Walter Russell, who came to Virginia in 1608 was a "Doctour of Physicke" and Lawrence Bohun, De la Warr's physician, had the same degree. Pott, who succeeded Bohun as physician-general of Virginia in 1621, came recommended as a Master of Arts well-practiced in surgery and physics.

After the Company's charter was annulled, few physicians or surgeons with the advanced medical degrees came to Virginia. Some of the persons, however, who practiced medicine in Virginia without medical degrees had acquired skills and knowledge in Europe or England before coming to the New World.

Patrick Napier who came to Virginia about 1655 as an indentured servant and subsequently had a large medical practice, probably learned his profession in England or on the Continent, as might have Francis Haddon, another who came under terms of indenture and who later, also, had a considerable medical practice. To these two examples of persons with training and experience acquired prior to their arrival in America might be added the similar experiences of John Williams and John Inman.

Medical knowledge and practices brought over from England were cross-fertilized with the European even in the New World. While the majority of newcomers were Englishmen, French, German, and other European physicians and surgeons came to Virginia. These European medical men appear, in general, to have prospered in Virginia and were anxious to become naturalized "denizens to this country."

George Hacke, born in Cologne, Germany, settled in Northampton County, Virginia, in 1653 and was known as a doctor and practitioner of medicine.

He was typical of the European-trained medical man settling in Virginia in becoming naturalized and in leaving a considerable estate, including thousands of acres of land. Little is known of his medical activities and interests except that he was summoned to treat the victim of a duel and that he left a large library which probably included volumes on medicine.

Paul Micou, a young French physician who seems to have acquired his education abroad, settled on the shores of the Rappahannock river, near a place afterward called Port Micou, during the last decade of the seventeenth century. Cultured and educated, he soon won prominence and wealth as a physician (and surgeon), attorney, and merchant. County records in Virginia make numerous references to suits brought by him for nonpayment of fees, suggesting an extensive practice.

Because so many of the doctors and surgeons of seventeenth-century Virginia are given only slight mention in the records, it is impossible to know whether, in most cases, they had acquired their skills and educations before coming to Virginia, or even whether they were born in the New World. Nor is it known how many young men born in Virginia went back to England or Europe to study medicine; a reference made by the famous English surgeon, John Woodall, indicates that a Virginian named Wake may have studied under him in London.

Within the Virginia county records, however, can be found evidence indicating that a common method of learning the profession was by apprenticeship. One interesting example of the contract between apprentice and surgeon survives in the records of Surry County, Virginia; made in 1657, it bound Charles Clay to Stephen Tickner, surgeon, for a term of seven years. Clay swore to serve his master in whatever surgical or medical duties he was assigned, and Tickner promised to use his best skill and judgment to teach his apprentice whatever he knew of the art. Another contract for apprenticeship was made between Richard Townshend and the London Company's well-known Dr. Pott. This relationship included a breach of contract that occurred not infrequently between master and apprentice: Townshend argued in court that Pott was not teaching him the "art & misterye" for which he was bound.

As an apprentice, the would-be physician or surgeon could gather herbs for his master and assist him in treating the sick. If the apprentice could read, or if the master would teach him, then the novice could study the medical books in the doctor's library. Not only were volumes on medicine available, but in the libraries of the better-educated medical men, the apprentice could also familiarize himself with other fields of learning.

Dr. Pott had a reputation for knowing Latin, Greek, and Hebrew, and must have imparted much of his learning to Richard Townshend, his apprentice.

Such would seem to be the case in view of the facts of Townshend's life. He became an apprentice to Pott in 1621 and by 1636 he was a member of the colony's highest political body, the council, and at the time of his death he possessed a considerable amount of land. In a day when schooling was hard to come by, apprenticeship to an educated man held great advantages.

Unfortunately catalogues of the libraries of medical men have not survived. There is proof, however, that physicians and surgeons did not neglect opportunities to collect volumes on medicine published in England and Europe. If utilized, these books could have helped offset the lack of a formal education in a university or medical school. Dr. Henry Willoughby of Rappahannock County, Virginia, left forty-four books on "phisick" in his estate. Dr. John Holloway, a leading physician of Accomack County, Virginia, from 1633 until his death in 1643, left thirteen books on surgery and medicine, all in English or Latin. Dr. Henry Andrews of York County had twenty books in Latin on medicine.

A great number of Virginians—some of them prominent—who did not practice medicine had, nonetheless, large collections of books on the subject. This would indicate that many persons resorted to medical treatment without the help of a professional. With fees high, distances great, and well-trained doctors scarce, self-reliance is not surprising. Many planters and their wives must have made a superficial study of medicine; certainly the mistress of the house visiting sick servants and slaves is a familiar historical picture.

Among the medical books in such libraries were volumes on the general subjects of medicine (physick) and surgery, anatomy, gout, scurvy, distillation, and natural magic. Common in the libraries of the laymen were books recommending specific drugs for various symptoms of diseases. The long title of one volume in a Virginia library read, "Method of physick, containing the causes, signes, and cures of inward diseases in man's body from the head to the foote. Whereunto is added the forme and rule of making remedies and medicines, which our physitions commonly use at this day, with the proportion, quantity, and names of each medicine."

The importance of medical volumes to the lay library is indicated by the inclusion of two in the supplies provided by a London agent for a Virginia plantation in 1620-21. William S. Powell, in a recent study of books in Virginia before 1624, found that the agent chose *The French Chirurgerye*, published in English in 1597, and the *Enchiridion Medicinae*, first published in 1573.

In spite of medical books, the apprenticeships, training in Europe or England, and the demand for medical services despite a high fee, it is possible to overestimate the competence of the seventeenth-century Virginia doctor even by the standards of his own century. An observation made by William

Byrd II early in the next century tends to reduce the stature of the medical man.

"Here be some men," Byrd wrote, "indeed that are call'd doctors; but they are generally discarded surgeons of ships, that know nothing above very common remedys. They are not acquainted enough with plants or other parts of natural history, to do any service to the world...." Byrd may have been prejudiced by his father who, although believing himself facing death, still did not call a physician.

CHAPTER FIVE

Conclusion

PORTRAIT OF A SEVENTEENTH-CENTURY VIRGINIA PHYSICIAN

Historical evidence does not support Byrd's description of the typical physician as a discarded ship's surgeon. In contrast, the physician, whatever his competence may have been, emerges from the sources as a respected member of the colony who, besides his medical practice, engaged in farming sizable holdings of land and took part in the civic life of the colony. His private life was not unlike that of the other planters who enjoyed some wealth and professional standing. The reputable surgeon, who could also supplement his income from farming, probably enjoyed an existence not unlike that of the physicians, considering that the distinction between them in the New World was slight.

Dr. Blanton, in his volume on medicine in Virginia, created a lively portrait of what he imagines from his researches to be the seventeenth-century Virginia doctor. The doctor is seen:

dressed in knee breeches and jerkin, perhaps adorned with periwig and cap; not given to church-going, but fond of ale, horse-racing and cuss words; husband of a multiparous wife; owner of a log cabin home or at best a frame cottage which he guarded with gun, pistol and scimitar; his road a bridle path and his means of conveyance a horse or boat ... reading ... by candle light, without spectacles; writing with a goose quill pen; sitting on a rough stool or bench; eating at a crude table from pewter dishes, without fork or table knife; having no knowledge of bath tubs; keeping his clothes in trunk or chest; sleeping, night-capped, on a flock bed in a bedroom shared by others; dividing his time, which he measured with hour-glass and sundial, among medicine, politics and farming; often in court, often a justice, member of Council or Burgesses, and subject, like his neighbors, to military service.

SUMMARY

Englishmen and Europeans planted Virginia in the New World and brought the Old World's medical knowledge and medical practices with them. In Europe and England, the seventeenth century witnessed the perfection of new and scientific theories in medicine—it was the century of Harvey—but little original and fruitful in the field of practice—Dr. Sydenham might be considered an exception.

In Virginia, the prior occupants had accumulated medical knowledge, too, and the Indians practiced in a manner not completely unlike that of the whites: bloodletting, purging, and sweating (all to the end of relieving the body of ill humors or morbid matter). The Indians, however, did not believe it right or good to impart their knowledge to the layman, Indian or European; therefore, cross-fertilization between the two schools of medicine was limited.

In planning for the colony, the London Company took into account that health would influence the fortunes of the new settlement. The Company warned the original settlers to choose a site in a healthful location, but the colonists elected Jamestown Island which was low and moist. Provided two surgeons by the Company, the original settlers needed not only more surgeons but physicians as well: the surgeons could treat the wounds, sprains, and breaks of a military-colonizing expedition, but physicians were needed to meet conditions that developed in Jamestown.

In subsequent boatloads of settlers, physicians did come—and some were well-trained and experienced—but the small number that arrived during the period when the London Company administered the colony (1606-24) could not meet the demands of disease and famine. During the first summer more than one-half the original settlers perished: during the Starving Time (1609-10) the population dropped from 500 to 60 and in the spring these 60 almost abandoned Virginia. A deadly combination of new environment, famine, and epidemic disease, such as typhoid, played a major part in determining the course of events during the first two decades of the colony's life, and near death.

After Virginia became a Crown colony, famine and disease no longer influenced affairs so greatly, not because of the wise administration of the Crown, but because the colonists had better learned what was necessary to cope with health conditions in the New World. No longer did they consider disease and famine minor threats compared to those from the Indians and Spaniards. They planned their ocean voyages so as to arrive in the fall and thus avoid the dread summer sickness while still too weak from the voyage to resist it; they located their outer settlements on higher and drier land, at the end of the century even moving their capital to Williamsburg, known for its temperate and healthful climate.

The physicians and surgeons, however, who came later in the century were not as distinguished as their earlier counterparts. As the century passed, many men trained by apprenticing themselves in Virginia. Whether immigrant or indigenous, the medical men used orthodox European techniques: they bled and purged, sweated and dispensed drugs, to obtain these ends. Some of the drugs were native to Virginia and the colonists exported them for a profit, but the more expensive—and efficacious—had to be imported. There is evidence that the level of medical excellence in Virginia lowered during the century; many of the planters avoided the expensive visits and drugs, even passing laws to regulate fees and chastise lax and inadequate practitioners.

Women, clergymen, and laymen all treated the sick and wounded of the period, with the women especially active as midwives; with the clergy producing such an outstanding medical man as the Reverend John Clayton; and with the laymen acquiring enough information, perhaps from a few medical books, in order to practice, themselves, in case a doctor were unavailable or undesired.

ACKNOWLEDGEMENTS AND BIBLIOGRAPHICAL NOTE

Dr. Wyndham B. Blanton kindly gave permission for the use, in the preparation of this booklet, of his definitive and authoritative volume on the history of seventeenth-century Virginia medicine. Dr. Blanton's work—based on extensive research in the sources—has proved of great value, but he should not be held responible for any weaknesses in this essay, as the author assumes full responsibility. The author also wishes to take this opportunity to express his appreciation for the numerous suggestions and improvements made by his wife who spent many hours assisting in the preparation of the manuscript.

The books and articles that proved most helpful were:

Allen, Phyllis, "Medical Education in 17th Century England," *Journal of the History of Medicine and Allied Sciences*, I (January, 1946), 115-143.

American History Told by Contemporaries. Edited by Albert B. Hart. New York and London, 1908-1909. 4 vols.

Beverley, Robert, *The History of Virginia*.... (Reprinted from the author's 2d rev. ed., London, 1722.) Richmond, 1855.

Blanton, Wyndham B., *Medicine in Virginia in the Seventeenth Century*. Richmond, 1930.

Brown, Alexander, *Genesis of the United States*. Boston and New York, 1890. 2 vols.

Castiglioni, Arturo, *A History of Medicine*. Translated from the Italian and edited by E. B. Krumbhaar. New York, 1941.

Chitwood, Oliver P., *A History of Colonial America*. New York, 1948.

Craven, Wesley F., *Dissolution of the Virginia Company: the Failure of a Colonial Experiment*. New York, 1932.

Southern Colonies in the Seventeenth Century, 1607-1689. Baton Rouge, 1949.

Duran-Reynals, Marie Louise, *The Fever Bark Tree*. New York, 1946.

Garrison, Fielding H., *An Introduction to the History of Medicine*.... Philadelphia, 1929.

Narratives of Early Virginia, 1606-1625. Edited by Lyon G. Tyler. New York, 1907.

Packard, Francis R., *History of Medicine in the United States*. New York, 1931. 2 vols.

Sigerist, Henry E., *American Medicine*. Translated by Hildegard Nagel. New York, 1934.

Smith, John, *Travels and Works*. Edited by Edward Arber. Edinburgh, 1910. 2 vols.

Tyler, Lyon G., "The Medical Men of Virginia," *William and Mary College Quarterly*, XIX (January, 1911), 145-162.

Wertenbaker, Thomas J., *The First Americans, 1607-1690*. New York, 1944.

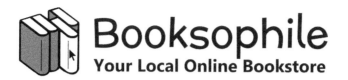

Booksophile
Your Local Online Bookstore

Buy Books Online from
www.Booksophile.com

Explore our collection of books written in various languages and uncommon topics from different parts of the world, including history, art and culture, poems, autobiography and bibliographies, cooking, action & adventure, world war, fiction, science, and law.

Add to your bookshelf or gift to another lover of books - first editions of some of the most celebrated books ever published. From classic literature to bestsellers, you will find many first editions that were presumed to be out-of-print.

Free shipping globally for orders worth US$ 100.00.

Use code "Shop_10" to avail additional 10% on first order.

Visit today
www.booksophile.com